GW01018106

Models of Care in Maternity Services

Models of Care in Maternity Services

Edited by
**Tahir Mahmood, Philip Owen,
Sabaratnam Arulkumaran**
and **Charnjit Dhillon**

© 2010 Royal College of Obstetricians and Gynaecologists

First published 2010

All rights reserved. No part of this publication may be reproduced, stored or transmitted in any form or by any means, without the prior written permission of the publisher or, in the case of reprographic reproduction, in accordance with the terms of licences issued by the Copyright Licensing Agency in the UK [www.cla.co.uk]. Enquiries concerning reproduction outside the terms stated here should be sent to the publisher at the UK address printed on this page.

Registered names: The use of registered names, trademarks, etc. in this publication does not imply, even in the absence of a specific statement, that such names are exempt from the relevant laws and regulations and therefore free for general use.

Product liability: Drugs and their doses are mentioned in this text. While every effort has been made to ensure the accuracy of the information contained within this publication, neither the authors nor the publishers can accept liability for errors or omissions. The final responsibility for delivery of the correct dose remains with the physician prescribing and administering the drug. In every individual case the respective user must check current indications and accuracy by consulting other pharmaceutical literature and following the guidelines laid down by the manufacturers of specific products and the relevant authorities in the country in which they are practising.

The rights of the Authors have been asserted by them in accordance with the Copyright, Designs and Patents Act, 1988.

ISBN 978-1-906985-38-7

A machine-readable catalogue record for this publication can be obtained from the British Library [www.bl.uk/catalogue/listings.html]

Published by the **RCOG Press** at the
Royal College of Obstetricians and Gynaecologists
27 Sussex Place, Regent's Park
London NW1 4RG

Registered Charity No. 213280

RCOG Press Editor: Jane Moody
Index: Cath Topliff
Design & typesetting: FiSH Books, London
Printed in the UK by Bell & Bain Ltd, 303 Burnfield Road, Thornliebank, Glasgow, G46 7UQ, UK

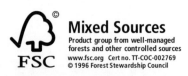

Mixed Sources
Product group from well-managed
forests and other controlled sources
www.fsc.org Cert no. TT-COC-002769
© 1996 Forest Stewardship Council

Contents

About the authors

Walaá Al-Safi FRCOG
Consultant Obstetrician and Gynaecologist
Rotherham NHS Foundation Trust, South Yorkshire, UK

Sabaratnam Arulkumaran KBE FRCOG
Head of Obstetrics and Gynaecology
St George's University of London, UK
President (at time of writing)
Royal College of Obstetricians and Gynaecologists, London, UK

Sonia Barnfield MRCOG
Senior Registrar in Obstetrics and Gynaecology
Southmead Hospital, Bristol, UK

Kirstyn Brogan MRCOG
Consultant Obstetrician
Ayrshire Maternity Unit, Crosshouse Hospital, Scotland, UK

Alan Cameron FRCOG
Consultant in Maternal Fetal Medicine
Southern General Hospital, Glasgow, UK

David Churchill FRCOG
Consultant Obstetrician/Director of Governance
New Cross Hospital, Wolverhampton, UK

Charnjit Dhillon
Director of Standards
Royal College of Obstetricians and Gynaecologists, London, UK

Tim Draycott MRCOG
Consultant Obstetrician
Southmead Hospital, Bristol, UK

Leroy Edozien FRCOG
Consultant Obstetrician and Gynaecologist
St Mary's Hospital, Manchester, UK

Corelia Hagmann FRCPCH
Clinical Lecturer
UCL Elizabeth Garrett Anderson Institute for Women's Health,
London, UK

Jane Hawdon FRCPCH
Consultant Neonatologist
UCL Elizabeth Garrett Anderson Institute for Women's Health,
London, UK

Alix Henley
Improving Bereavement Care Team
Sands, the stillbirth and neonatal charity, London, UK

Mary Hepburn FRCOG
Consultant Obstetrician and Gynaecologist
Princess Royal Maternity Hospital, Glasgow, UK

Mervi Jokinen
Practice and Standards Development Advisor
Royal College of Midwives, London, UK

Donna Kirwan MPhil
National Projects Officer
NHS Fetal Anomaly Screening Programme, UK National Screening
Committee, UK

Justin Konje FRCOG
Professor of Obstetrics and Gynaecology and Honorary Consultant
Leicester General Hospital, Leicester, UK

Sailesh Kumar FRCOG
Consultant and Senior Lecturer in Maternal and Fetal Medicine
Queen Charlotte's and Chelsea Hospital, Imperial College, London, UK

Rachel Liebling MRCOG
Consultant in Fetal Medicine and Obstetrics
St Michael's Hospital, Bristol, UK

Boon H Lim FRCOG
Consultant Obstetrician and Gynaecologist
Hinchingbrooke Healthcare NHS Trust, Cambridgeshire, UK

Tahir Mahmood FRCOG
Consultant Obstetrician and Gynaecologist
Forth Park Maternity Hospital, Scotland, UK
Vice President, Standards
Royal College of Obstetricians and Gynaecologists, London, UK

Elizabeth McGrady FRCA
Consultant Anaesthetist
Glasgow Royal Infirmary, Glasgow, UK

Lyn McIntyre RN
Programme Lead
NHS East of England, Cambridge, UK

Heather Mellows FRCOG
Consultant Obstetrician and Gynaecologist and Professional Advisor
Partnerships for Children, Families and Maternity, Department of
Health, London, UK

Jo Modder MRCOG
Consultant Obstetrician
UCL Elizabeth Garrett Anderson Institute for Women's Health,
London, UK

Jessica Moore MRCOG
Consultant in Obstetrics and Gynaecology
St George's Hospital NHS Trust, London, UK

Edward Morris FRCOG
Consultant Obstetrician and Gynaecologist
Norfolk and Norwich University Hospital, Norwich, UK

Osric Navti MRCOG
Consultant in Maternal Fetal Medicine
Leicester General Hospital, Leicester, UK

Caroline Overton FRCOG
Consultant Obstetrician and Gynaecologist
St Michael's University Hospital, Bristol, UK

Timothy Overton FRCOG
Consultant in Fetal Medicine and Obstetrics
St Michael's University Hospital, Bristol, UK

Philip Owen MRCOG
Consultant Obstetrician and Gynaecologist
Princess Royal Maternity Unit, Glasgow, UK

Roshni Patel MRCOG
Consultant Obstetrician
Chelsea and Westminster NHS Foundation Trust, London, UK

Helen Scholefield MRCOG
Consultant Obstetrician
Liverpool Women's Hospital, Liverpool, UK

Judith Schott
Improving Bereavement Care Team
Sands, the stillbirth and neonatal charity, London, UK

Gordon Smith FRCOG
Professor of Obstetrics and Gynaecology
Cambridge University, Cambridge, UK

Baskaran Thilaganathan FRCOG
Professor of Fetal Medicine
St George's Hospital NHS Trust, London, UK

Suzanne Truttero
Midwifery Advisor
Department of Health, London, UK

Vishal Uppal FRCA
Registrar in Anaesthesia
Glasgow Royal Infirmary, Glasgow, UK

Acknowledgement

We would like to record our appreciation for the hard work of Maria Finnerty, who provided administrative support.

Abbreviations

A&E	accident and emergency
AAGBI	Association of Anaesthetists of Great Britain and Ireland
AchR	acetylcholine receptor
ACOG	American College of Obstetricians and Gynecologists
AOI	Adverse Outcomes Index
ASW	Antenatal Screening Wales
ATSM	Advanced Training Skills Module
BASHH	British Association of Sexual Health and HIV
BMI	body mass index
CASE	Consortium for the Accreditation of Sonographic Education
CCT	Certificate of Completion of Training
CE	European Conformity
CEMACH	Confidential Enquiry into Maternal and Child Health
CEMD	Confidential Enquiries into Maternal Deaths
CEM T21	Condensed Education Module for Trisomy 21 (Down syndrome)
CHD	congenital heart disease
CMACE	Centre for Maternal and Child Enquiries
CNST	Clinical Negligence Scheme for Trusts
CPD	continuing professional development
CQC	Care Quality Commission

CQUIN	Commissioning for Quality and Innovation
CRL	crown–rump length
CTG	cardiotocography
DH	Department of Health
DoSySP	Down Syndrome Screening Programme
DQASS	Down Syndrome Screening Quality Assurance Support Service
ECG	electrocardiogram
FASP	Fetal Anomaly Screening Programme
FGR	fetal growth restriction
FHR	fetal heart rate
GMC	General Medical Council
GP	general practitioner
HIE	hypoxic ischaemic encephalopathy
ICP	integrated care pathway
IVF	in vitro fertilisation
LeSSon	lead screening sonographer
MOEWS	modified obstetric early warning system
MOM	multiples of the median
MOMS	Management of Myelomeningocele Study
MRI	magnetic resonance imaging
NCT	National Childbirth Trust
NHS	National Health Service
NHSLA	National Health Service Litigation Authority
NICE	National Institute for Health and Clinical Excellence
NICU	neonatal intensive care unit

NPSA	National Patient Safety Agency
NSC	National Screening Committee
NSF	National Service Framework
NT	nuchal translucency
OAA	Obstetric Anaesthetists' Association
PCT	primary care trust
QA	Quality Assurance
QIPP	quality, innovation, productivity, prevention
RAG system	red, amber, green system
RCM	Royal College of Midwives
RCoA	Royal College of Anaesthetists
RCOG	Royal College of Obstetricians and Gynaecologists
RCPCH	Royal College of Paediatrics and Child Health
RSI	repetitive strain injury
SGA	small for gestational age
SHA	strategic health authority
SIGN	Scottish Intercollegiate Guidelines Network
SLE	systemic lupus erythematosus
TSH	thyroid-stimulating hormone
TUMSG	Trust Ultrasound Multidisciplinary Screening Group

Preface

This book is all about improving the quality of care in maternity services. The individual chapters reflect the fact that the main drivers for improvement are clinical effectiveness and increasing patient expectations. In each area of practice described, there is recognition that the appropriate clinical response to these drivers is service organisation. This book will help clinicians to take responsibility not only for managing individual patient conditions but also for developing services that meet patients' needs.

Clinical developments will only come about if clinicians take the initiative to ensure that improvements happen. This book demonstrates that much can be achieved within current resources and without the need for major additional expense. Different approaches are demonstrated but the key issue is the patient pathway, with the underlying philosophy of continuous improvement in quality.

Clinical leadership is the key to success. There is increasing evidence that obstetricians and gynaecologists are more than equal to the task and recognise the satisfaction that derives from being associated with clinical development and improvements in the quality of care for women. Trainees, clinicians, managers and commissioners of services will find this book of practical value and there should be a copy on the shelves of every hospital obstetric unit.

Professor Sir Sabaratnam Arulkumaran
President (at time of writing)
Royal College of Obstetricians and Gynaecologists

CHAPTER 1
Setting the scene

Sabaratnam Arulkumaran and Tahir Mahmood

Introduction

Maternity services in the UK enjoy high-quality, safe service, yet there is room for improvement. The Healthcare Commission survey carried out 3 years ago highlighted that 89% of women are satisfied or are more than satisfied with the care provided.[1] Maternal mortality in the UK is 13/100 000 and 50% of cases are from direct causes. Substandard care has been identified in a number of cases. The clinical spectrum of cases seen in current labour wards appears to be different from that seen 50 years ago and the same is true for the causes of maternal mortality and morbidity. Maternal mortality from cardiac disease 40 years ago was mainly attributable to rheumatic heart disease. In the late 1990s, death was due to congenital heart disease. In the first decade of the 21st century, increasing numbers of deaths are from acquired heart disease such as myocardial infarction. This change may be because of background factors such as obesity, increasing age, associated conditions such as hypertension and diabetes and an increasing number of immigrant women presenting with undiagnosed cardiomyopathies. The Confidential Enquiry into Maternal Deaths 2003–2005 indicated that nearly 33% of mothers who died were in the obese category.[2] An additional dimension that has come to light is that more pregnancies are presenting with complex social factors; for example, more maternal deaths are seen in women whose children are in care. Psychiatric disease is one of the leading indirect causes of maternal death.

Although we have to recognise and pay more attention to these issues, there is a demand to improve the quality of care that will provide emotional satisfaction to the couple, their relatives and the caregivers. Attention has to be paid to improving the quality of care for the vast majority of the 700000 mothers who give birth each year in the UK. This in itself will improve not only quality but also safety for all mothers. The models of care we design have to follow the principles that they are easily available, accessible, acceptable and affordable. They should also have safety as the backbone on which to build better quality. It should also be remembered they have to be affordable and achieved through efficient working, as quality does not necessarily require additional large sums of money. All the quality improvement initiatives will succeed only when clinicians take the lead for efficient use of resources to deliver the agreed goals.

Pregnancy is a period of physical and psychological stress. Care should be designed from the prepregnancy stage through to pregnancy, intrapartum care, postnatal care and long-term follow-up for the selected few who had maternal illness during pregnancy. The mothers who had diabetes or hypertension in pregnancy have an increased chance of developing these conditions in later life and the continuum of care should be extended in such a way that they are followed up by their family practitioners regularly so that their quality of life is improved and their lifespan is extended. This is important not only for the individual woman but also for her family.

There should be a major drive towards improving the social issues of smoking, drinking, housing and the possibility of work to improve quality of life. In addition to public health and medical issues, we must provide high-quality maternity care and the fundamental to this is treating women with respect and dignity. This, we believe, can be achieved by one-to-one care, by having a named midwife or a group of midwives in a single team, to enable the woman to have access to the named midwife or her colleagues in that team. Standards of care need to be established and agreed by the professionals and the consumers, adherence to which should result in high-quality safe care.

▉ Standards for maternity care

The Royal College of Obstetricians and Gynaecologists (RCOG), the Royal College of Midwives (RCM), the Royal College of Paediatrics and Child Health (RCPCH) and the Royal College of Anaesthetists (RCoA) have jointly published *Standards for Maternity Care*.[3] Standards are defined from prepregnancy to transition to parenthood, supplemented by general standards related to the provision of high-quality care. Best-quality, safe care can be provided by adherence to these standards. There should be an annual audit to identify adherence to the expected standards. The maternity standards used by the Clinical Negligence Scheme for Trusts (CNST) to support the work of the NHS Litigation Authority[4] are heavily influenced by the documents produced by the RCOG and other important documents such as the *Saving Mothers' Lives* report.[2] This working arrangement provides us with leverage to develop strategies to implement the standards of care published by the RCOG.

In the document *High Quality Care for All*, Lord Darzi and his team set out an ambitious vision to improve quality by the development of quality matrices.[5] The report recommended the use of clinical dashboards to monitor clinical outcomes related to clinical activity and patient-related outcomes. The Maternity Dashboard, a part of the RCOG Good Practice advice series, helps to fulfil the needs of the clinical dashboard.[6] This dashboard has been used in many NHS trusts, who have found it useful to identify shortcomings so that action can be taken to improve care. Chapter 20 in this book deals with the details of the maternity dashboard.

Clinical governance

The principles of clinical governance should be embedded into our local quality framework. Clinical governance is a mechanism whereby essential elements needed to provide the best care are regularly monitored with the aim of constantly improving the quality of current performance. The maternity dashboard displays the seven pillars that underpin clinical governance (Figure 1.1).

1. **The work place** should have adequate capacity to provide antenatal, intrapartum and postnatal care. It should have the required equipment, which should be up-to-date and checked at the beginning of each shift to make sure that it is in working order. The environment should be safe, clean and user-friendly.
2. **The workforce** should be adequate to provide the required services in a timely and friendly manner. Workforce issues related to staffing in the labour ward (medical, midwifery and support staff) are dealt with in the RCOG document *Safer Childbirth*.[7] For good-quality care in an obstetric unit there should be one midwife for every 28 deliveries. There should be 168 hours of consultant presence if the total number of deliveries is over 6000/year. In units that deliver over

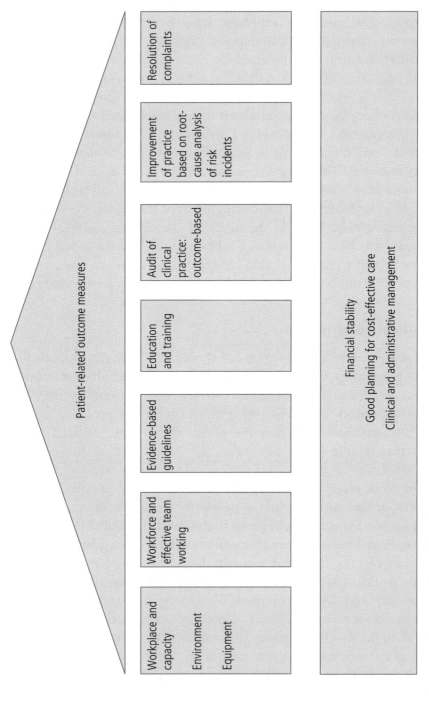

Figure 1.1 The seven pillars of clinical governance

5000 births/year we should work towards this target. Analysis of the incidents reported to the National Patient Safety Agency (NPSA) suggests that risk incidents are associated with the unavailability of seniors and not enough staff to provide care.[8] These two factors are associated with most risk incidents. It is also known that a fair number of medical litigation cases and adverse outcomes tend to happen outside working hours and over the weekends. Labour and delivery can happen at any time of the day or night or the weekends, hence the need to have a sufficient number of senior staff and midwives to tackle these problems in an obstetric unit.[9]

3. **Evidence-based guidelines** should be used to provide best individualised care by multiprofessional teams within the constraints of the resources and facilities available. It is important to ensure that women's views are respected.

   The essential components of evidence-based medicine are distilled as clinical guidelines by the National Institute for Health and Clinical Excellence (NICE) and as Green-top Guidelines by the RCOG. The Green-top Guidelines have been assessed to be of high quality by an independent panel of assessors at NHS Evidence and now feature on the website of NHS Evidence. These guidelines are accessible freely to all clinicians, midwives, healthcare planners and commissioners of services. We are justly proud of this achievement as this should encourage all clinicians to use guidelines in order to influence commissioning.

   Individual hospitals may like to adapt these guidelines into a one- or two-page flowchart that can be followed easily. It is important for the guidelines to be up-to-date and available as a hard copy in addition to being on the internet. Midwives, obstetricians, anaesthetists and paediatricians who provide maternity care should have ready access to these guidelines. This helps the various professionals to understand each others' roles and to work as a team.

4. **Education and training** are important to keep professionals up-to-date and practising according to the guidelines. One of the CNST requirements is to monitor multiprofessional training. Multiprofessional training sessions focusing around key areas such as interpretation of cardiotocographic tracings, review of adverse outcomes and regular obstetric drills enable better team work, starting with good communication without hindrance. The challenge for clinical directors is to run these sessions regularly in their units and also to facilitate attendance of those working on night shifts.

5. **Clinical audit**: auditing our practice will lead to improvement in care. Neither NICE nor the RCOG has regulatory powers to force individual trusts to audit, although some areas are required by the CNST to be audited regularly. Individual trusts must develop local strategies to regularly review clinical practice to deliver evidence-based care and undertake audits to evaluate whether their units are practising what is recommended in evidence-based guidelines and whether it is resulting in good clinical outcomes. Auditable standards on different aspects of maternity care are provided in the *Standards for Maternity Care* document.[3] The consultant-in-charge of each area of maternity care should consider auditing the recommended standards as part of the quality improvement process. Each consultant and the midwifery matron-in-charge of separate subsections of their maternity unit should target one or two auditable standards each year with the hope of improving the quality of care in different areas of clinical practice. In this way, each unit could go through most of the auditable standards over a 3–5-year cycle. Such a practice is likely to lead to high-quality, safe care.

6. **Monitoring risk incidents** for the frequency and magnitude of risk is essential. Most maternity units have risk management teams. Incident reporting to identify risk is based on certain trigger factors formulated by the RCOG.[10] Studying the risk incidents and providing recommendations based on root-cause analysis should improve safety and quality. These recommendations should be disseminated to all staff to avoid recurrence of similar risk incidents. A newsletter in the form of *Risky Business* should be available every month from the risk management team for the rest of the staff to know what risk incidents have occurred and how they could have been avoided.

7. **Complaints** from women and staff should be treated seriously. Response to complaints should be within a recognised timeframe and the team should put in place measures that will minimise the recurrence of similar incidents leading to complaints. This should be high on the agenda of clinical and midwifery directors. Complaints should be categorised according to whether they are caused by system error or by professional behaviour in the form of poor or hostile communication or attitude. There should be zero tolerance of complaints related to behaviour or communication. The reputation of a unit can be damaged by the misbehaviour of a small minority of staff resulting in recurring

complaints. Appropriate disciplinary action should be taken if it is the same individual(s) who is/are at the centre of the complaints.

The above-mentioned seven pillars constitute the clinical governance framework and should be taken seriously if one is to improve the safety and quality of maternity care, whether it is in a stand-alone or co-located midwifery unit or an obstetric unit.

Summary

These seven pillars should stand on the foundation of the professional commitment of those who work in maternity units, who should cooperate with each other to enhance team work that will deliver compassionate care that builds confidence about the quality and safety of care among the women who use the service. The foundation should be supported by adequate financial resources and clinical and managerial support. These elements in the foundation will enable the seven pillars to stand strongly. Attention to the foundation and the seven pillars will improve patient-related outcome measures, akin to the roof on the seven pillars of the building.

The professional bodies have a responsibility to help individuals and institutions to provide the high-quality care we expect for our own kith and kin. Adherence and provision of care described in *Standards for Maternity Care* is a preventative measure to avoid unsafe incidents and to promote high-quality care. The maternity dashboard gives a monthly review of the clinical workload, staffing levels, staff training, clinical outcomes, interventions, number of clinical risk incidents and complaints. This monitoring process will help us to identify the parameter at risk and enable us to take appropriate action before safety and quality are compromised. Clinical indicators in the dashboard provide continuous monitoring. If there is a reduction in the number of women admitted to the intensive care unit and the number of postpartum hysterectomies following massive postpartum haemorrhage, one could also expect fewer women to be transfused. If this reduction can be demonstrated month by month and year by year, it suggests that the obstetricians, midwives, anaesthetists and haematologists have worked effectively as a team. Similarly, if the number of unexpected admissions of term babies to the neonatal intensive care unit is reduced, it suggests that there has been concerted action by the midwives, obstetricians and neonatal paediatricians to carefully follow guidelines in electronic fetal monitoring. Such measurement should reassure us of our practice or hint at the need for improvement.

■ The way forward

Models of Care in Maternity Services highlights good practices as perceived by our contributors and covers many general principles discussed in this chapter. The content of the chapters reflects available evidence and what is observed in good units. The book highlights issues arising from the *Standards for Maternity Care* and *Safer Childbirth* documents. Passing on the technological know-how of good practice can improve safety and quality. Sir Liam Donaldson, Chief Medical Officer for England, who has visited a number of units inspecting different services, often said that there are centres of excellence in a sea of mediocrity. He advocated that we have to build bridges from these centres of excellence to the other centres. His observations were not about whole units; even in a perceived less well-performing unit there are two or three subunits providing excellent service.

With the deepening financial crisis in the world, there will never be enough new money available to invest in the NHS in the UK. There are already considerable pressures on NHS staff to derive efficiency and cost containment to deliver a high-quality clinical service. It is reassuring to note that quality initiatives are at the top of the NHS agenda. This vision will be achieved by the development of quality indicators that would underpin Commissioning for Quality and Innovation (CQUIN). Furthermore, the QIPP initiative (quality, innovation, productivity, prevention) will help to embed evidence-based clinical practice to reduce variations in clinical practice, as well as making it cost-effective.[11] All these initiatives for driving quality in women's health services are most welcome. We believe that this book follows that philosophy and will help to increase quality and safety in maternity services.

■ References

1. Healthcare Commission. *Women's Experiences of Maternity Care in the NHS in England: Key Findings from a Survey of NHS Trusts Carried Out in 2007*. London: Commission for Healthcare Audit and Inspection; 2007 [www.cqc.org.uk/publications.cfm?fde_id=7962].
2. Lewis G, editor. *Saving Mothers' Lives: Reviewing Maternal Deaths to Make*

Motherhood Safer 2003–2005. The Seventh Report of the Confidential Enquiries into Maternal Deaths in the United Kingdom. London: CEMACH; 2007 [www.cmace.org.uk/Publications/CEMACH-Publications/Maternal-and-Perinatal-Health.aspx].

3.   Royal College of Anaesthetists, Royal College of Midwives, Royal College of Obstetricians and Gynaecologists, Royal College of Paediatrics and Child Health. *Standards for Maternity Care. Report of a Working Party.* London: RCOG Press; 2008 [www.rcog.org.uk/womens-health/clinical-guidance/standards-maternity-care].

4.   NHS Litigation Authority. Clinical Negligence Scheme for Trusts: Maternity Clinical Risk Management Standards Version 1 2010/11 [www.nhsla.com/News/ #{A0A8EE5C-A421-4925-AD44-6DF4E3ED8DDC}].

5.   Department of Health. *High Quality Care For All: NHS Next Stage Review Final Report.* CM 7432. London: TSO; 2008 [www.dh.gov.uk/en/publicationsandstatistics/publications/publicationspolicyandguidance/DH_085825].

6.   Royal College of Obstetricians and Gynaecologists. *Maternity Dashboard: Clinical Performance and Governance Scorecard.* Good Practice No 7. London: RCOG; 2008 [www.rcog.org.uk/womens-health/clinical-guidance/maternity-dashboard-clinical-performance-and-governance-score-card].

7.   Royal College of Obstetricians and Gynaecologists, Royal College of Anaesthetists, Royal College of Midwives and Royal College of Paediatrics and Child Health. *Safer Childbirth: Minimum Standards for the Organisation and Delivery of Care in Labour.* London: RCOG Press; 2007 [www.rcog.org.uk/womens-health/clinical-guidance/safer-childbirth-minimum-standards-organisation-and-delivery-care-la].

8.   National Patient Safety Agency. Fetal and Maternal Compromise Incidents Reported to NPSA Between June 2006 and May 2007. London: NPSA; 2007.

9.   Royal College of Obstetricians and Gynaecologists. *Responsibility of the Consultant-on-Call.* Good Practice No. 8. London: RCOG Press; 2009 [www.rcog.org.uk/ responsibility-of-consultant-on-call].

10. Royal College of Obstetricians and Gynaecologists. *Improving Patient Safety: Risk Management for Maternity and Gynaecology.* Clinical Governance Advice No. 2. London: RCOG Press; 2009 [www.rcog.org.uk/improving-patient-safety-risk-management-maternity-and-gynaecology].

11. Department of Health. *The NHS Quality, Innovation, Productivity and Prevention Challenge: An Introduction for Clinicians.* London: DH; 2010 [www.dh.gov.uk/en/ Publicationsandstatistics/Publications/PublicationsPolicyAndGuidance/DH_113806].

CHAPTER 2

Developing and implementing a local maternity services strategy: the clinical director's role

David Churchill and Tahir Mahmood

Key points

✓ When developing a local maternity services strategy, involve all interested parties (patients, staff, and commissioners) and take information from regulators and standard-setting bodies.
✓ Patients expect and value safety above everything else.
✓ When implementing change, form multidisciplinary teams around the processes that need changing and encourage those with expertise to step forward and become leaders.

▓ Introduction

Being a clinical director is a multifaceted role. The clinical director is expected to be a leader, strategist, negotiator, arbitrator, manager and doctor. When developing and implementing a local maternity services strategy, all aspects of the role will be active at some time. Following the development of a strategy, the clinical director will have to persuade colleagues to work towards its implementation.

Much of the work of a clinical director carries a large element of common sense and much of this chapter will be familiar territory to the experienced clinical director. However, the principles outlined will be recognised as fundamental, even if, over time, the detail changes. The first part of the chapter describes how to build a strategy and the second part the essential elements of its implementation.

Developing a maternity services strategy

What is a strategy? Put simply, it is a long-term plan but, in putting the plan together, it is important to know the final objectives and direction of travel.

The views of many groups and individuals will need to be considered when drawing up a local maternity services strategy. Broadly, they can be categorised into three elements:

- the patients or users of the service
- the commissioners, policy makers and regulatory bodies
- the professionals who deliver the service.

Careful consideration must be given to the views expressed by each group so that the final document receives broad agreement.

Perspective of women using maternity services

Women who use maternity services form the most important interest group. When gathering and collating their views it will be necessary to ensure that the whole spectrum of the local population is consulted. A strategy that is unduly influenced by one particular pressure group or another will be biased and will lead to unexpected clinical risks for segments of the population.

Two significant surveys of women who use maternity services in the UK were published in 2008: the Healthcare Commission published *Towards Better Birth* and the Picker Institute carried out a survey that informed the King's Fund report on safety in maternity services.[1-3] These are useful as starting points before embarking on a local consultation. The results of both surveys provide the clinical director with valuable information to consider.

The Healthcare Commission report was set against the background of several adverse reports arising from investigations into a number of maternity services.[1] The Commission's concerns were that some trusts had staffing levels well below the average, indicating that they may have been inadequate; consultant obstetricians were not spending the recommended amount of time on labour wards, as set out by their professional bodies; in-service training was poorly attended; continuity of care was inadequate; and recommendations for antenatal care, especially for those at risk, were not being followed.

The Commission surveyed both staff and users to gain evidence for the report. More than 26 000 women responded to the survey and the Healthcare Commission reported that 80% or more of the women questioned rated the care they received as good, very good or excellent. There were areas in need of improvement: 20% of women rated their postnatal care as either fair or poor.

There was also a degree of variation between trusts. In the trust with the least favourable rating, only 67% of mothers reported their care during labour and birth as good or better. This compared with a level of 97% in the trust with the most favourable ratings. Two other aspects of care that received unfavourable comment from women were the provision of information about their condition and its management and their involvement in decisions about their care.

In the second survey, the Picker Institute interviewed 31 recently pregnant women from diverse ethnic and socio-economic backgrounds. This survey showed, unsurprisingly, that women expect safe care as a basic standard. When those surveyed were asked which elements of the maternity service demonstrated that it was of a high quality and provided safe care, they selected the following five areas:

- one-to-one midwifery care in labour
- appropriate staffing levels
- team working and staff who engendered confidence
- patients who felt respected
- high-quality environment.

The bond with the midwife throughout labour was fundamental to the experience of those surveyed. The reassurance provided by skilled professionals who kept them informed and involved in the decision making mattered more than anything else. When the relationship worked well, even serious complications were faced with confidence.

When the women were asked what gave the impression of unsafe care, the answers highlighted the following four areas:

- low staffing levels
- poor monitoring
- inadequate and conflicting information
- being left alone in labour.

The women referred to labour as a natural process but also accepted that childbirth carried inherent risks. All but one chose hospital rather than a home birth, feeling safer in the knowledge that emergency facilities were readily available.

Both of these surveys warrant reading in full to distil their important messages. However, the views of women using local services will need to be canvassed by each department for the strategy to be relevant to their needs. Questionnaires, surveys and bodies such as maternity services liaison committees will provide the necessary information.

While we all strive to provide the services our patients want and need, financial constraints limit what can be achieved in the short and medium terms. It is therefore the role of the clinical director and their team to prioritise the developments arising out of the strategy. Safety of patients and protection of the vulnerable must guide this process. After this has been done it is useful to get the perspective of the patients using the service once again.

Policies standards and regulation

All maternity services strategies will have to take into account government policies, standards set by professional bodies and limits set by regulators. Fortunately, the last two areas overlap considerably, but sometimes government policy will present a challenge, pushing services to develop in ways the professionals see as counterproductive. The clinical director will need to navigate a sensible course through these areas.

National policy

Following a broad consultation with professionals and the public, the Department of Health published *High Quality Care for All*.[4] This document summarised the challenges facing the healthcare system:

- rising patient expectations
- demands driven by changing demographics
- continuing development of the information society
- advances in treatment
- changing nature of disease
- changing expectations of the healthcare workplace.

The blueprint for the future of the NHS included the commissioning of services for wellbeing and prevention, tackling obesity, reducing smoking and a national campaign to make care safer. The role of the National Institute for Health and Clinical Excellence (NICE) was expanded to develop quality standards.

Choice has been a common theme running through many government policies. *Maternity Matters* gave a national choice guarantee with four promises:[5]

- choice on how to access maternity care
- choice on the type of maternity care
- choice on the place of birth
- choice in postnatal care.

This document set the context for improvement at the local level. Commissioners and providers of maternity services must ensure that in planning services for the future the requirements of the local population are taken into account. Maternity services must also support the national target of reducing health inequalities in infant mortality and life expectancy at birth.

The theme of choice was developed further in the National Service Framework for Children's and Maternity Services, which emphasised the need for 'women-centred individualised care'.[6]

Fortunately, both patients and policy makers recognise that choice is constrained by issues of safety. Maternity services strategies must therefore be balanced with safety standards as laid down by professional bodies to protect the mother and baby.

Professional standards and safety

Until recently, professional standards and safety involved a significant paper chase to gather all the appropriate information. The four Royal Colleges involved in the provision of maternity services (obstetrics and gynaecology, midwifery, anaesthetics and paediatrics) have synthesised, from 50 source documents, all the standards relating to maternity services into one useable document, *Standards for Maternity Care*.[7] Together with clinical pathways of care, the report details the dimensions required for support and governance of maternity services. Each set of standards is accompanied by a group of audit indicators to use when measuring compliance. This is an excellent reference document and starting point for all professionals involved in delivering high-quality maternity services. However, developments are occurring rapidly in the area of clinical standards and patient safety. It will therefore be necessary to periodically scan the relevant websites for the most up-to-date information. Apart from the Colleges, NICE provides a sound evidence base to inform current practice, and the NHS Institute for Improvement and Innovation website (www.institute.nhs.uk) provides advice and access to the various tools available with which to monitor patient safety.

Staff views

The third element of strategy development is to obtain the views of all staff groups involved in delivering the service. As with the patients' contribution, it is important to have the whole spectrum of staff contribute to the strategy. While there have been national surveys of NHS staff, these are no substitutes for obtaining views locally. While this may be an arduous process, it is vital if the strategy is to become a dynamic document to ensure that those delivering the service make the required changes to their service in the interest of patients.

Once the strategy has been agreed, a plan of action will need to be drawn up to bring about its implementation.

Putting the strategy into action

Implementation of the strategy's action plan will require clear leadership from the clinical director and the senior team. There will be a need for persistence, determination and an ability to adapt to changing circumstances. A case study demonstrating the development and the implementation strategy of a first-trimester combined screening test for Down syndrome in the unit is included as Box 2.1.

Developing and leading a team

During the development of the strategy, enthusiasts and activists will have emerged throughout the process. Their expertise should be harnessed in the implementation stages. Playing to people's strengths by using their expertise in their chosen areas of interest will pay huge dividends. This does not mean that they will all step forward and volunteer. Many may require

Box 2.1 The implementation of a first-trimester combined screening test for Down syndrome

Drivers for change

Locally, the provision of NHS screening for Down syndrome rested with the second-trimester, serum screening, 'triple' test. First-trimester screening was only available through the private sector. Consequently, the majority of the local population were denied the opportunity of a superior screening test at an earlier gestation. This ran counter to the local and national commitment to provide clinical services equitably. In addition, the National Screening Committee published its directive for Down syndrome screening standards. It recommended, as the preferred option, that services implemented first-trimester combined screening by 2010.

The team

A project team was assembled. The members were:

- the consultant obstetrician responsible for antenatal screening
- the antenatal screening coordinator midwife
- a fetal medicine ultrasonographer midwife
- a superintendent sonographer
- the midwifery matron for antenatal and outpatient services
- the directorate operational manager
- the head of midwifery
- the regional screening coordinator.

The aim

The aim was to provide universal access to first-trimester combined screening for Down syndrome.

Service redesign

Preliminary discussions were held with the staff involved in the provision of the Down syndrome screening service. The reasons for the proposed changes were explained and all committed to redesigning the care pathway and introducing first-trimester screening.

An exercise was then performed to examine gaps in capacity to introduce the change. It was clear that, in bridging the gap, the redesign would need to encompass the antenatal clinic pathway. The opportunity was therefore taken to redesign and integrate both pathways, with the joint aims of introducing the new screening test and reducing waiting times in the antenatal clinic.

With the help of the hospital's service redesign team the pathway was redesigned using 'lean' methodology. The service areas involved included community midwifery, the antenatal clinic, the fetal medicine unit, maternity ultrasound and administration. Following this exercise and the reconstruction of the care pathway, several factors critical to the success of the project were identified by the team.

The laboratory where the risk assessment was carried out agreed to issue letters for all women who were low-risk, informing them of their result. The high-risk results were handled as before, by the laboratory faxing the fetal medicine department, where appropriate action was taken.

Training

- There was a need to extend the roles of the antenatal clinic maternity support workers, training them in phlebotomy and collecting essential patient data. The training was delivered by the haematology department.
- All ultrasonographers were trained to measure the nuchal translucency by staff from the Fetal Medicine Foundation.
- Administration staff were trained in the new requirements for appointments within the gestational parameters for the test. A fast-track system was developed for women who presented to their community midwife late in the first trimester.
- Community midwives were all trained in the information to give to women about Down syndrome screening in general. This was to prepare women who wanted screening for the first-trimester test or, if they were not suitable, for the second-trimester screening test.

Information

- Patient information was revised.
- Antenatal referral letters were redesigned. A box was introduced for women who chose the Down syndrome screening programme.
- A new referral form was designed to include the data on the nuchal translucency measurement and the patient's weight, ethnic group and smoking status.

Capacity and resources

- The ultrasound scanning capacity was also examined using the principles of 'lean'. Basing the calculations on a 100% uptake, there was a shortfall of 35 scan appointments each week. One day of a whole-time equivalent ultrasonographer was required above the current complement of staff to meet the shortfall.
- The antenatal clinic had a shortfall of two maternity support workers to meet the phlebotomy needs of the new screening programme.
- The extra funding required for the staffing shortfall was found by reaching maternity Clinical Negligence Scheme for Trusts level 3 and receiving a rebate on the insurance premium and internal departmental savings.
- The extra cost of £2/sample, for serum testing, was funded by the primary care trust, which committed to funding the service in the long term.
- The total extra recurrent funding was £50,000/year.

Audit

- The take-up rate of testing for Down syndrome was monitored for each test method. Before the start of the new programme, the Down syndrome screening rate was 60% of all women booked. In the first 3 months of the new programme it increased to 78%. In the second 3 months it fell back to 69%. Of those women choosing Down syndrome screening, 82% underwent the first-trimester test and 18% the second-trimester serum screening. Patient satisfaction was high.

- Approximately 230 women/month have the first-trimester testing and the screen-positive rate is 1.5%, well within the National Screening Committee's target for test performance.
- Two complaints were received. These women were high-risk and had been appropriately managed but still received 'low-risk' letters. They were sent directly from the laboratory, where the error occurred. This problem has now been corrected.

Outcome

- The new pathway for antenatal clinic and antenatal screening worked well. The resources required were as predicted and there have been positive benefits in other areas of clinical activity. Training the maternity support workers to a higher level has increased their job satisfaction and they have used their skills to help in other areas of activity, such as glucose tolerance testing and organising emergency blood tests.
- Women welcomed the new service and staff were happier being able to provide equity for all women.
- The amount of training in the new system of information giving for community midwives was underestimated. This resulted in the antenatal screening coordinator having to provide a second and third round of training sessions before they were all happy.

Conclusion

The new screening pathway was introduced successfully to the satisfaction of the women accessing the service. A more equitable service was provided. The roles of maternity support workers were extended, having beneficial effects in other areas of activity. The pathway through the antenatal clinic was also streamlined, reducing waiting times.

encouragement and persuasion. It is therefore the role of the clinical director to spot the talent.

These leaders will need teams to deliver areas of work. Teams are more successful when formed around a process they all understand. Multidisciplinary teams should be grouped around the work streams. Each team must be given clear objectives with defined outcomes. Vague instructions or ill-defined objectives will lead to a breakdown in the team structure as individuals will start to pursue their own agendas. Above all else, the clinical director will have to put their trust in those delivering specific work streams. Each team must be given the power to act and resolve problems for themselves. This will enhance their feeling of ownership and encourage the team to greater efforts.

Methodologies of change management

It is easy to be cynical about the methodologies of change management. They are unscientific and rely on linear thinking. There have been many movements over the years and there is overlap among them all. Nevertheless, they do offer a framework within which teams can operate and think about the services they provide. Systematically assessing the processes involved in the provision of a service, seeing the processes from the viewpoint of the patient, cutting out waste and improving the safety and quality of the care delivered are principles that everyone can agree upon.

Most success can be achieved by taking a practical approach, focusing on the processes involved in delivering care rather than abstract ideas of culture and participation. The right culture will develop out of participation in the redesign, as long as the values of the workplace are strong. This requires commitment from the senior team. The various models can be distilled into several stages:

Stage 1   The senior team has to gain commitment for change from the whole department.

Stage 2   Out of stage 1, the senior team must develop and then share the future strategy. A statement of change must define the boundaries for the department.

Stage 3   Critical success factors need to be developed. They define the direction and success criteria or end products of the process. The result should be a balanced set of deliverables.

Stage 4   Key performance indicators or targets must be chosen and the data required to monitor the process defined.

Stage 5   The core service delivery processes that deliver the critical success factors must be understood. It may be necessary to break these down into subprocesses.

Stage 6   Improvement teams must then set to work on the specific processes to make changes to improve the quality and/or safety of the service provided to the patients.

Stage 7 The key performance indicators and outcome measures must be assessed to determine the success of any change made. If the outcomes are not those that are expected, a period of analysis is required to identify the problems to ensure success.

There are several useful texts in the area of change management, some of which have examples of change introduced in the healthcare setting of the UK.[8–10]

By applying these techniques to the processes of medical care it is possible to improve the quality of service for all patients. It is important to review any implemented changes through systematic audit to ensure that they are having their desired effects and not causing any problems for patient safety.

Training and education

Changes brought about by the introduction of a new service strategy will expose the need for further training and education of certain members of staff. The teams leading the change will identify these needs themselves. They may in fact go further than first envisaged. Their enthusiasm must be encouraged and the clinical director should ensure that all is done to meet the training needs. The result will be a more stable and dynamic workforce, which will pay huge dividends to the department in the future, enabling it to adapt more readily to a changing environment.

Staff receiving training in new skills should be encouraged to pass on their learning to the rest of the workforce. This is especially important in the arena of patient safety and is vital in keeping risks to a minimum.

Resolving conflicts

There will inevitably be conflicts within and between teams. In these situations, the clinical director will have to assume the role of arbitrator. The best agreements are those that satisfy the concerns of both sides. When this is not possible and after hearing all the arguments it is important for the clinical director to make a clear decision on the way forward. The decision and the reasons for arriving at it should be expressed clearly to all concerned.

Governance and risk management

The introduction of change will always have some unexpected consequences that may be counterproductive to the strategy. Recognising these problems at an early stage will minimise their detrimental impact. To recognise issues, the clinical director will need a mechanism for regularly monitoring key processes and outcomes. Staff must also be encouraged to report problems through an incident reporting system.

Knowledge and practice in governance and clinical risk management has grown over the last decade. While an in-depth analysis is beyond the scope of this chapter, it is worth drawing out two of the key elements and newer developments that can help the clinical director when introducing changes in a department.

All clinical directors will need information on a regular basis that informs them of the safety performance of their department. Often the amount of information can be daunting, but dashboards of key process and outcome indicators have been developed to aid their identification.[11] These dashboards act as early warning systems, alerting the observer when a particular process may be going out of control. During a period of change, a worthwhile exercise is to review the number and type of key indicators in the dashboard. It is often useful to add in some indicators for a period of time that cover the specific service area undergoing the most significant change.

Many dashboards have colour schemes to indicate the level of control, but these data can be further analysed in a simple way. Run charts and, in some instances, statistical process control charts will add an extra dimension to the information.[12] These charts are easy to construct and provide a visual representation of a trend. This is particularly useful when giving feedback on the effects of change on a system.

The most valuable component of a risk management system is incident reporting and it remains so during the implementation of strategic change. Encouraging the staff to recognise problems and report incidents is key to producing a sustainable service change. No system is ever perfect, but solving problems as soon as they arise will prevent major difficulties in the future. Clinical directors should actively seek out staff and ask about any problems that they may have encountered and the solutions they developed. Teams solving problems for themselves will build resilience into a system, but the clinical director must be prepared to help them by bringing in other expertise when the solution to the problem lies outside their control.

◼ Summary

Putting together a local maternity services strategy is not easy. It requires a degree of soul searching from maternity departments to identify their weaknesses. The views from all the interested parties must be gathered and reflected in a balanced way in the final document. The commitment of those delivering the maternity services must be wholeheartedly in support of the strategy and its implementation. Nevertheless, the benefits of a successfully implemented strategy will be tangible for patients and long lasting for the department.

◼ References

1. Healthcare Commission. *Towards Better Births. A Review of Maternity Services in England*. London: Commission for Healthcare Audit and Inspection; 2008 [www.cqc.org.uk/publications.cfm?fde_id=625].
2. Rowe R, Magee H, Heron P, Quigley M, Askham J, Brocklehurst P. *Women's Experience of Antenatal Screening: Are there social and ethnic inequalities in access to antenatal screening for Down's syndrome?* Oxford: NPEU and the Picker Institute; 2007.
3. Magee H, Askham J. *Women's Views about Safety in Maternity Care. A Qualitative Study*. London: King's Fund; 2008 [www.kingsfund.org.uk/applications/site_search/ ?term=Women%E2%80%99s+Views+about+Safety+in+Maternity+Care.+A+qualita tive+study&searchreferer_id=2&submit.x=31&submit.y=4].
4. Department of Health. *High Quality Care for All: NHS Next Stage Review Final Report*. Cm7432. London: The Stationery Office; 2008 [www.dh.gov.uk/en/publica-tionsandstatistics/publications/publicationspolicyandguidance/DH_085825].
5. Department of Health; Partnerships for Children, Families and Maternity. *Maternity Matters: Choice, Access and Continuity of Care in a Safe Service*. London: DH; 2008 [www.dh.gov.uk/en/Publicationsandstatistics/Publications/ PublicationsPolicyAndGuidance/DH_073312].
6. Department of Health. *National Service Framework for Children, Young People and Maternity Services Standard 11: Maternity Services*. London: DH; 2004 [www.dh.gov.uk/en/Publicationsandstatistics/Publications/PublicationsPolicyAndGui dance/Browsable/DH_4094336].
7. Royal College of Anaesthetists, Royal College of Midwives, Royal College of Obstetricians and Gynaecologists, Royal College of Paediatrics and Child Health. *Standards for Maternity Care. Report of a Working Party*. London: RCOG Press; 2008 [www.rcog.org.uk/womens-health/clinical-guidance/standards-maternity-care].
8. Oakland, JS. *Total Organizational Excellence: Achieving World-class Performance*. 2001. 2nd ed. Oxford: Butterworth-Heinemann; 2001.
9. Stahr H, Bulman B, Stead M. *The Excellence Model in the Health Sector: Sharing Good Practice*. Chichester: Kingsham Press; 2000.
10. Jackson S. *Using the EFQM Excellence Model Within Healthcare: A Practical Guide to Success*. Chichester: Kingsham Press; 2001.

11. Royal College of Obstetricians and Gynaecologists. *Maternity Dashboard: Clinical Performance and Governance Scorecard*. Good Practice No. 7. London: RCOG; 2008 [www.rcog.org.uk/womens-health/clinical-guidance/maternity-dashboard-clinical-performance-and-governance-score-card].
12. NHS Institute for Innovation and Improvement. Safer care: improving patient safety [www.institute.nhs.uk/safer_care/safer_care/safer_care_-_home_page_2.html].

CHAPTER 3

Prepregnancy services for women with social needs

Mary Hepburn and Kirstyn Brogan

Key points

✓ Prepregnancy care for women with social needs should enable women to protect and control their fertility and to ensure any pregnancies are intended and optimally timed for good medical and social outcomes.

✓ Prepregnancy care for women with social needs is essential to promote social as well as physical stability and wellbeing prior to conception.

✓ Prepregnancy care for women with social needs should include general health promotion including advice about folic acid supplementation.

✓ Prepregnancy care can improve outcomes in high-risk pregnancies regardless of whether the high-risk status is of medical or social aetiology.

✓ Women who are socially disadvantaged do not seek advice through routine health channels. Multidisciplinary agencies already providing services for such women should be trained in needs assessment and delivery of basic components of prepregnancy care and should collaborate with reproductive healthcare services to ensure routine provision of prepregnancy care for all women with whom they are in contact.

✓ Complementary services including information, education and social and health care should be provided for socially disadvantaged men and partners of socially disadvantaged women.

▥ Introduction

There has long been recognition that poverty, social exclusion and social problems are associated with poorer health.[1] There are consequently increased adverse outcomes of pregnancy among women with social problems.[2] Disadvantage, social problems and associated lifestyles have an overall negative impact on health, but there may also be specific problems for mother and baby. For example, problem drug or alcohol use can lead to bloodborne virus infection, liver damage, cardiac valvular damage or thromboembolic disease; prostitution can lead to sexually transmitted infection and violence or abuse resulting in physical injuries, mental illness and addiction. While these in turn can increase morbidity among the babies, treatment of the problems is not without its risks; for example, drugs used to treat bloodborne viruses, mental illness and problem drug use can also cause ill health in the neonate. The adverse health effects of social problems are often long-term and extend into adulthood.

Across the social spectrum, many pregnancies are unplanned. However, while pregnancies among socially disadvantaged women are often unplanned, they are not necessarily unintended or unwelcome. The need for prepregnancy services in the management of women with pre-existing medical conditions such as diabetes has long been acknowledged. The impact of socio-economic deprivation and social problems caused by or exacerbated by deprivation can be at least as severe as that caused by maternal medical problems. Recognition that such women need specialised maternity care has been slow to develop: recognition that they need specialised prepregnancy care is still widely unrecognised. This is particularly disappointing, since many women with such problems are already in contact with medical and social services. This affords an ideal opportunity to engage with women, to discuss their reproductive plans and to provide them with the necessary services to enable them to control and protect their fertility so that any pregnancies they may have are planned and timed for optimal medical and social outcomes.

It is important to recognise that women with socially related problems will have the same desire to have children as their nondisadvantaged peers. They will also aspire to have healthy babies that they are able to parent adequately. It is important not to prejudge the issue and to work with such women towards a positive goal, recognising that any preconception health and social input will be worthwhile and will maximise the outcome of any pregnancy that occurs.

▮ What women want

Routine prepregnancy health promotion is not generally available, but there are a number of surveys demonstrating women's desire for this to be introduced.[3,4] Prepregnancy care is also acceptable to health professionals, but this is often within a GP setting and targets women who are motivated.[5]

There are no published reports of prepregnancy care being routinely offered to women with additional social needs. There is, however, a desire for specialist care. Experience in many centres nationally and internationally has demonstrated that, if provided with appropriate specialist services, socially disadvantaged women and women with special needs will attend early and regularly for antenatal care. Hepburn and Elliott highlighted the features that made a service acceptable to this group of women, the most important being staff awareness and knowledge about the relevant social issues together with a nonjudgemental approach.[6] They also demonstrated that 46% of women were currently using illicit drugs. It was observed that there was a reduction in illicit drug usage over the course of pregnancy. With preconception advice this may be further decreased. Similarly, medication for other problems such as mental illness could be reviewed and social circumstances assessed and stabilised.

Since most women with special needs would be unaware of the potential benefits, they would be unlikely to seek out prepregnancy care and might decline such care if it were offered without adequate explanation. However, experience in Glasgow has confirmed that such women welcome prepregnancy care if provided by a specialist reproductive health service as a routine part of their management within services already dealing with their other problems.

■ National guidance and clinical guidelines

There is currently no national guidance on prepregnancy care for the UK population. In 2006, the USA published recommendations and guidelines on preconception care for all women, but these guidelines do not specifically address the needs of socially disadvantaged women.[7]

Some women with pre-existing medical conditions such as diabetes and adult congenital cardiac disease receive prepregnancy care within their specialist clinics. Other women who are well motivated will seek advice from their general practitioner or another health professional. These women are seldom from vulnerable groups. The introduction of folic acid supplementation preconception has reduced the number of fetal neural tube defects, but this prevention relies on women being informed of the benefits of folic acid supplementation preconception and being motivated to take it. Women with social needs are often poor attenders at GP practices and other health provision sites.

The *Saving Mothers' Lives* report[2] discusses service delivery for women with drug and alcohol misuse and also notes that these women may have other social needs. One of the recommendations of this report is that clear, relevant and complete information on social problems, including substance misuse, should be provided by GPs in referral letters to the antenatal care team and these potentially high-risk pregnancies should be fast-tracked to an integrated service between addiction and maternity services, ideally supervised by an obstetrician. Women should not be managed in isolation but by maternity services that are part of a larger multi-agency network. Guidelines addressing the issue of substance misuse during pregnancy recognise the impact and associated social problems on the health and social outcomes of pregnancy.[8,9] These guidelines do not acknowledge that addressing these issues once the woman is already pregnant is often too late. Appropriate health and social care, education and support prior to pregnancy may reduce substance misuse, improve maternal health and stabilise social issues leading to improved outcomes.[10,11]

■ Service modelling and care pathways

Women with high-risk pregnancies need obstetrically led care embedded in maternity services. Thus, for example, women with diabetes receive obstetrically led antenatal care provided by a multidisciplinary team within a maternity setting. Similarly, women with high-risk pregnancies as a consequence of social problems are not suitable for midwifery-only care (although, as in the medical high-risk model, a great deal of care can be delivered by midwives within the multidisciplinary team). Such women should receive obstetrically led care from a multidisciplinary team and while input may be provided in a number of settings, management of their pregnancy should be based within a maternity setting.

Outside of pregnancy, however, reproductive health care, while vitally important, does not have such a central role and can be opportunistically delivered within other services attended by the women. For example, women attending addiction, psychiatric or mental health services, women who suffer homelessness, violence or abuse, women who are seeking asylum and many other vulnerable women involved with a variety of agencies are readily accessible and would benefit from reproductive healthcare and planning.

Where such care is provided for vulnerable women, it is often provided as an optional opt-in service that women must choose to have. However, even if women are routinely offered the option of prepregnancy counselling and care, they may not know what is on offer or be aware of the potential benefits. Raising awareness is therefore necessary among service providers as well as service users; many services and agencies working with disadvantaged, socially marginalised or vulnerable women are ideally placed to routinely provide prepregnancy care to all women who enter the service. Such prepregnancy care should include information and advice about pregnancy planning together with reproductive health care (including screening for sexually transmitted infections and cervical cytology) and effective contraception to enable women to defer pregnancy.

Special issues related to service delivery

While the service should be provided within non-reproductive healthcare – or even non-healthcare – services, it is important that those providing the care work in close collaboration with the host service, functioning as and perceived by the women as part of that service. They should also either be an integral part of the service providing maternity care or maintain close liaison with maternity services, with reproductive health care provided, and perceived by the women to be provided, as a continuum. The women should receive integrated health and social care with reproductive planning informed by all aspects of their health and social problems and management. Vulnerable women can be very mobile and contact with services may be interrupted without notice. It is therefore essential not only to adopt an opportunistic approach and deliver care within another service but to do it at the earliest opportunity, since delay on the part of either women or services may result in loss of the opportunity.

There may be overlap between health and social problems and, for example, women with HIV infection may receive input from a wide range of services. Such women may be regarded as medically rather than socially high-risk. Their need for prepregnancy care may be regarded as the remit of services for women at medically high risk, but is often not addressed in that context; moreover, they may have social problems that make them attend erratically for care or they may be mobile for reasons outside their control, as in the case of dispersion of asylum seekers. Some duplication of service provision by different services will be justified, but there is also a need for close collaboration to maximise the effectiveness of service provision.

Compromises may sometimes be necessary to ensure that women do not miss out on care; for example, it may be inappropriate to adhere rigidly to standard protocols on initiation of contraception with regard to menstrual cycle. This is particularly true for women who may have been amenorrhoeic for many months because of problem drug use, poor nutrition or another feature of their lifestyle. Ultimately, the priority is to ensure that women receive appropriate care.

Training

A number of initiatives have explored the need to incorporate education and training on health inequalities into both undergraduate and postgraduate curricula. On a national level, the Academy of Medical Royal Colleges Academy Health Inequalities Forum has developed a common curricular component to provide this for a range of healthcare professionals.[12] While health inequalities are already addressed in the training of relevant non-healthcare professionals, teaching on the links between social and health issues needs further development. There is also a need to raise awareness among non-reproductive healthcare workers, both health and non-health, of the need for and benefits from prepregnancy advice and treatment to promote optimal timing of pregnancies and their role in facilitating this.

All reproductive healthcare professionals must be trained and able to take a full social history in both the prepregnancy and maternity setting. While aspects of social history have been incorporated into the antenatal booking history (such as routine enquiry about domestic abuse and routine enquiry about problem drug and alcohol use) as well as topics perceived as intrusive or potentially stigmatising (such as routine offer of antenatal HIV testing), these issues are usually addressed in isolation. While the knowledge may be topic-specific, the same skills are required in each case and a unified approach should be taken with regard to training in taking a social history.

There is also a need for multidisciplinary training for relevant health and social staff. Shared documentation of core information is essential, but training is necessary to enable staff to record such information in a generic way to ensure essential information is shared without disclosing irrelevant medical details. While staff must operate within appropriate professional boundaries, they must also be aware of wider issues and areas of overlap. In particular, healthcare staff must be aware of child protection issues, their responsibility in this area and the need to provide health care informed by social circumstances and possible child protection concerns.

Staffing and manpower planning

Women with social problems also have health problems and need complex multidisciplinary care. Provision of such prepregnancy care to a potentially mobile population is challenging but extremely cost-effective. Much of current service provision is not mainstream but is often funded from specific short-term budgets allocated to individual social problems (such as problem drug and alcohol use, criminal justice, prostitution, homelessness). It is essential to recognise that acceptance of services by this group of women may take time and interruption in service provision can be very detrimental, so their reproductive health care should be provided as a mainstream service with continuity among different aspects of care. As in the case of women at medically high risk, the skill mix within such a service should reflect women's needs. Provision of reproductive health care, including prepregnancy care, for women with social problems should be incorporated into strategic planning and reflected in staffing levels and skill mix.

Audit

The following are appropriate auditable standards.

- Evidence of women being given prepregnancy care within multidisciplinary settings: proportions of women attending services (such as addiction, mental health, learning disability, homelessness) who have received prepregnancy care and proportions of pregnant women with these problems who have received prepregnancy care.
- Training of non-health professionals (for example, within addiction, mental health and learning disability services) in reproductive health care for women with social problems: awareness of the need for and potential benefits of prepregnancy care and the ability to take a basic reproductive health history, to contribute to service provision and to promote uptake of specialist input by women.

- The number of women with social problems taking folic acid at the time of booking visit.
- The proportion of pregnant women with problem substance use involved with addiction services prior to pregnancy.
- Documentary evidence of contraceptive discussion and family planning within services working with women with social problems.
- The proportion of pregnant women with social problems who have used contraception prepregnancy and patterns of contraceptive use.
- The existence of protocols for prepregnancy counselling.

■ Future research

While the case has yet to be made for prepregnancy care for women at low risk of problems, there is a clear clinical need for prepregnancy care to be provided for women with social problems. Development of routine service provision is a priority and such services should be subject to audit as described. The issue of research in this field is currently not a priority but should be reviewed once service provision has been established.

■ References

1. Townsend P, Davidson N. *Inequalities in Health: The Black Report.* Harmondsworth: Penguin Books; 1982.
2. Lewis G, editor. *Saving Mothers' Lives: Reviewing Maternal Deaths to Make Motherhood Safer 2003–2005. The Seventh Report of the Confidential Enquiries into Maternal Deaths in the United Kingdom.* London: CEMACH; 2007 [www.cmace.org.uk/Publications/CEMACH-Publications/Maternal-and-Perinatal-Health.aspx].
3. Adams MM, Bruce FC, Shulman HB, Kendrick JS, Brogan DJ. Pregnancy planning and pre-conception counseling. The PRAMS Working Group. *Obstet Gynecol* 1993;82:955–9.
4. de Jong-Potjer LC, de Bock GH, Zaadstra BM, de Jong ORW, Verloove-Vanhorick SP, Springer MP. Women's interest in GP-initiated pre-conception counselling in The Netherlands. *Fam Pract* 2003;20:142–6.
5. Heyes T, Long S, Mathers N. Preconception care: practice and beliefs of primary care workers. *Fam Pract* 2004;21:22–7.
6. Hepburn M, Elliott L. A community obstetric service for women with special needs. *Br J Midwifery* 1997;5:485–8.
7. Johnson K, Posner SF, Biermann J, Cordero JF, Atrash HK, Parker CS, et al. Recommendations to improve preconception health and health care: United Sates. A Report of the CDC/ATSDR Preconception Care Work Group and the Select Panel on Preconception Care. *MMWR Recomm Rep* 2006;55(RR-6):1–23.

8. Hogg C, Chadwick T, Dale-Perera A. *Drug Using Parents: Policy Guidelines for Inter-Agency Working (England and Wales)*. London: Local Government Drugs Forum; 1997.
9. Scottish Executive. Getting our Priorities Right: Policy and Practice Guidelines for Working with Children and Families Affected by Problem Drug Use. Edinburgh: Scottish Executive; 2003.
10. De Regil LM, Fernandez-Gaxiola AC, Dowswell T, PeÒa-Rosas JP. Effects and safety of periconceptional folate supplementation for preventing birth defects (Protocol). *Cochrane Database Syst Rev* 2009;(3):CD007950. DOI: 10.1002/14651858.CD007950.
11. MRC Vitamin Study Research Group. Prevention of neural tube defects: results of the Medical Research Council Vitamin Study. *Lancet* 1991;338:131–7.
12. Academy of Medical Royal Colleges. Health Inequalities Forum. *Health Inequalities Curriculum Competency Project*. London: AOMRC; 2009 [www.aomrc.org.uk/ committees/academy-health-inequalities-forum.html].

CHAPTER 4

Access to early pregnancy care

Caroline Overton and Tahir Mahmood

Key points

✓ Policies should be in place for the management of early pregnancy problems.

✓ Policies should be in place to meet the national target of booking women before 12 completed weeks of pregnancy.

✓ Strategies should be in place to identify women with pre-existing medical conditions.

✓ Strategies should be in place to identify socially disadvantaged women to develop individualised antenatal care.

✓ Effective communication strategies should be in place to support women who do not speak English to improve access to services.

■ Introduction

Early pregnancy services should be modelled in such a way that they are accessible to deal with all the problems of early pregnancy, such as bleeding and medical conditions such as hyperemesis gravidarum, and also to facilitate routine antenatal care before the 12th week of pregnancy.

■ Why is antenatal care important?

Antenatal care provides an opportunity for screening and optimising maternal and fetal health for a successful pregnancy, health and wellbeing. In 1993, the Expert Maternity Care Group from the Department of Health released the *Changing Childbirth* report, which made explicit the right of women to be involved in decisions regarding all aspects of their antenatal care.[1] One of the priorities of antenatal care is to enable women to make informed decisions about their care, such as where they will be seen, who will undertake their care, which screening tests they will have and where they plan to give birth. The first contact with health care should also help to quantify social and medical determinants of poor obstetric outcome. Such a targeted approach would allow inter-agency support systems to be put in place according to individual needs.

The challenge for each service is to develop local information showing a strategy to respond to the local population's needs.

Service users' views

In a survey of maternity services in the NHS, just over 30% of recent mothers reported that they felt they had the option to choose where they received their antenatal care. With screening tests, however, 60% of mothers reported feeling that they had been offered a choice.[2] In this survey, the views of 1188 pregnant women were explored on their information needs through self-completed questionnaires. Fifty percent of the women reported that they would have liked additional information at their first antenatal appointment, with first-time mothers most likely to believe that they had been provided with too little information. Written sources of information were also highly valued.[2]

This survey also reported on what women would like to learn in antenatal classes.[2] The responses included:

- information on physical and psychological changes during pregnancy
- fetal development
- what will happen during labour and childbirth
- options during labour and childbirth
- how to care for themselves during this time
- possible complications
- how to care for the baby after birth.

An independent enquiry conducted by the King's Fund found that the overwhelming majority of births in England are safe but that some births are less safe than they could and should be.[3] Patient safety is related to quality of care. Thus, a risk management system should be in place for early identification of problems and the systems should be able to deal with them. As maternity services are mostly delivered by teams rather than individuals, effective team working is one of the most important drivers of improved safety. Team members providing early pregnancy care need to be aware of each others' actions and be ready to step in with support and assistance.

National guidance and clinical guidelines

The NICE antenatal care guideline (2003) recommended that booking with maternity services should take place before 12 weeks of pregnancy.[4] The two most recent Confidential Enquiries into Maternal Deaths, *Why Mothers Die 2000–2002* and *Saving Mothers' Lives*, have identified late booking as one of the risk factors for maternal deaths.[5,6] In each enquiry period, 20% and 17%, respectively, of the women who died from direct or indirect causes had booked for maternity care after 22 weeks of gestation. *Saving Mothers' Lives* recommended that maternity service providers should ensure that antenatal services are accessible and welcoming so that all women, including those who currently find it difficult to access maternity care, can reach them easily and earlier in their pregnancy.[6] Women should also have their full booking visit and hand-held maternity records completed by 12 weeks of pregnancy.

Rowe and Garcia characterised a group of women who booked late or had fewer antenatal care appointments who were mainly from the lower social strata and of non-white ethnic origin.[7] The National Service Framework specifies that 'maternity services are proactive in engaging all women, particularly women from disadvantaged groups and communities, early in their pregnancy'.[8]

In *Maternity Matters*, the Government committed itself to four national choice guarantees that would be available to all women by the end of 2009:[9]

- the choice of how to access maternity care
- the choice of type of antenatal care
- the choice of place of birth
- the choice of place of postnatal care.

This document also urged commissioners to understand what in their current services prevented women from seeking care early or maintaining contact with maternity services. Commissioners were urged to put plans in place to overcome these barriers by providing more flexible services at times and places that meet the needs of these women. The report further stated that the commissioners and providers involved in planning maternity services must take into account the challenges set out above and the diversity of the local population to ensure that the very best care is available to provide new parents and their babies with a better start to family life.[9]

Similarly, the Healthcare for London and Newborn Clinical Working Group emphasises local easy-to-access midwifery care and recommends that women's social and medical needs should be assessed at an early stage and then reassessed during their pregnancy.[10]

The Public Service Agreement Delivery Agreement 19 sets out one of its indicators of progress as: 'the percentage of women who have seen a midwife or a maternity healthcare professional for health and social care assessment of needs, risks and choices for 12 completed weeks of pregnancy'.[11]

Identification of language needs

Saving Mothers' Lives highlighted the rapidly changing nature of motherhood; more than 20% of women who had babies in the UK in 2005 were themselves born elsewhere and English was not their first language.[6] In this report, 34 women died from direct or indirect causes and all spoke little or no English. Five of these women suffered fatal domestic violence. Timmins reported that 'non-English speaking status' was a marker of a population at risk of decreased access and that language barriers can adversely affect quality of care.[12] *Why Mothers Die* recommended the development of systems and protocols for accessing appropriate inter-preters.[5] This report further recommends that 'enquiries about violence should be routinely included when taking the social history at booking or at another opportune point in the antenatal period'.[5] Therefore, depending upon the ethnic composition of the area, anyone providing maternity services should be able to call on qualified interpreters.

Number of antenatal visits

NICE recommended ten appointments for nulliparous women and seven for parous women for routine antenatal care.[4] *Saving Mothers' Lives* identified poor attendance at antenatal care as one of the risk factors for maternal deaths.[6] The Healthcare Commission used this NICE recommendation to develop its clinical focus indicators – 'women not receiving NICE recommended number of antenatal appointments' – in the assessment framework for its maternity services review.[13]

Obesity and the risks during pregnancy

Studies in the UK and the USA indicate that maternal obesity carries risks for the mother and the baby. Complications associated with obesity include increased risk of miscarriage, gestational hypertension, gestational diabetes, pre-eclampsia, thromboembolism, emergency caesarean section, induction of labour, postpartum haemorrhage, fetal death, neural tube defects, shoulder dystocia, fetal macrosomia and wound infection.[14] *Saving Mothers' Lives* identified obesity as a risk factor for maternal deaths and has recommended a target of 100% for recording the body mass index of all pregnant women attending for booking visit.

■ Quality indicators and quality accounts

High Quality Care for All sets out the quality agenda for the NHS, which will be supported by the development and measurement of quality indicators, a function led by NICE and overseen by the National Quality Board.[15] Quality accounts are a legal requirement for all providers of NHS healthcare from June 2010.[16] The framework for quality indicators is available on the NHS Information Centre website.[17] For commissioning purposes, the Department of Health has released a set of 200 quality indicators, including indicators for maternity and gynaecology services. These include 'booking for antenatal care less than 12 weeks of gestation'.[17] Such activities will be captured through clinical dashboards, which, in a simple graphical format, will inform the daily decisions that drive quality improvement.[18] The RCOG has been in the forefront of developing these tools.[19]

Fetal Anomaly Screening Programme

The Fetal Anomaly Screening Programme has set up various initiatives in the UK, such as internal quality control of screening assays, management of ultrasound soft markers and the publication of leaflets for parents and professionals on 12 conditions.[20] Their website (http://fetalanomaly.screening.nhs.uk) is a useful resource for patients and professionals to access information leaflets on various diagnostic tests used for screening.

Domestic violence

Maternity Matters clearly points out risks related to the domestic abuse of women.[9] A multisite evaluation of independent domestic violence advisors, *Safety in Numbers 2009*, studied 2500 women over 2 years across seven sites in England and Wales.[21] These women were suffering from severe, high-risk physical, emotional and sexual abuse as well as stalking and harassment. The independent domestic violence advisors systematically mobilised and targeted the resources of up to 15 agencies on their behalf. This report found that this abuse stopped completely in two-thirds of cases where there was intensive support and an independent domestic violence advisor service, including multiple interventions. The maternity services providers should be aware of the contents of this report.

Alcohol

Approximately 90% of women in Britain consume alcoholic drinks at least occasionally. Between 1980 and 2006, per capita alcohol consumption in the UK rose by 21%. The survey of women in Britain revealed that 8% of women aged 18–24 years had consumed at least 35 units of alcohol in the past week. This is defined as harmful drinking by the Department of Health and the Home Office. Women should therefore be advised that excess alcohol has an adverse effect on the fetus.[22–24]

■ Service modelling and care pathways

The model of care for all early pregnancy events should be composed around the women's journey (Figure 4.1). Early pregnancy loss before 12 weeks of gestation is a common event, causing a great deal of distress to women and their partners, and healthcare providers need to direct considerable resources to looking after these women and their families. There are currently over 200 active early pregnancy units in the UK. The RCOG has promoted evidence-based care models for the management of miscarriage and ectopic pregnancy.[25]

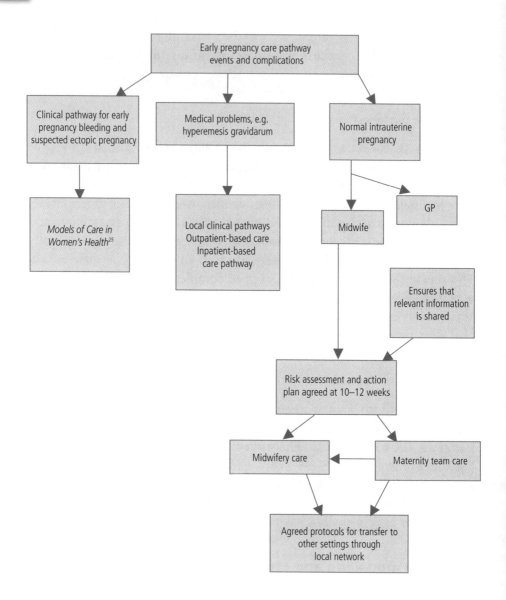

Figure 4.1 Access to early pregnancy care

Nausea and vomiting is now considered a normal physiological symptom of pregnancy in up to 90% of cases, except in a small proportion of women where persistent vomiting, dehydration and electrolyte disturbance could be a potentially life-threatening disease process. Severe nausea and vomiting is the third leading cause of hospitalisation during pregnancy.[26] It is important to have local care pathways in place for initial assessment, investigations for contributing causes and focused treatment.

Antenatal care pathway

This chapter will now focus on the objectives of engaging with women for an early antenatal booking appointment to identify their individual needs and develop individualised care plans that could make a difference in the outcome of their pregnancy (Box 4.1, Table 4.1).

Box 4.1 Women with special needs requiring inter-agency input

- Women from disadvantaged groups: learning and physical disabilities
- Women who are socially deprived
- Teenagers, unemployed, those in an unstable relationship
- Single parents
- Ethnic minority groups
- Women with complex medical and social histories
- Asylum seekers
- Women with a history of female genital mutilation

Table 4.1 Ascertainment of risk factors

Identification of risk	Screening programme
Past medical history of epilepsy, diabetes, cardiac disease	Down syndrome
Poor obstetric history	Neural tube defect
Severe pre-existing or past mental illness	Rubella
Obesity (body mass index >30)	Syphilis, HIV
Thromboembolic risk	Hepatitis
Lifestyle issues (smoking, drug misuse, alcoholism)	Haemoglobinopathies
Dietary issues	Rhesus programme
Domestic abuse, housing and social services support	

Women with uncomplicated pregnancy should be looked after by their midwife and GP. There should be continuity of care throughout the antenatal period and antenatal care should be readily and easily accessible. The environment in which antenatal appointments take place should enable women to discuss sensitive issues such as domestic violence, sexual abuse, psychiatric illness and illicit drug use. Care should take into account the individual needs of the pregnant woman (Box 4.2).

Box 4.2 Key standards for early pregnancy care

- Contact details for midwives should be easily accessible in the local population.
- Prepregnancy counselling and support should be provided for women of childbearing age with pre-existing serious medical or mental health conditions.
- All women who experience complications in early pregnancy should have prompt access to an early pregnancy assessment service.
- Women should have had their first full booking visit and hand-held maternity record completed by 12 weeks of pregnancy.
- Women with social needs and disadvantaged groups should receive adequate support through inter-agency arrangements.

Women should have had their first full booking visit and hand-held maternity record completed by 12^{+0} weeks of pregnancy. Women like to carry their own maternity care records. This can lead to increased feeling of control during pregnancy. It may also facilitate communication between the pregnant woman and the health professionals involved in her care.[27-29] Maternity service providers should ensure that antenatal services are accessible and welcoming so that all women, including those who currently find it difficult to access maternity care, can reach them easily and earlier in their pregnancy.

Special needs of women from abroad

All pregnant women from countries where women may experience poorer overall general health and who have not previously had a full medical examination in the UK should have their medical history taken and a clinical assessment made of their overall health, including a cardio-vascular examination at booking to look for an undiagnosed cardiac disease such as rheumatic valvular disease and cardiomyopathies.[5,6] This assessment should be performed by an appropriately trained doctor, who could be the woman's usual GP. Women from countries where genital mutilation or 'cutting' is prevalent should be sensitively asked about this during their pregnancy and management plans for delivery agreed during the antenatal period.[30]

Smoking cessation

Smoking is a significant modifiable cause of adverse pregnancy outcome in women and its dangers have been widely established, particularly low birth weight and preterm birth. The benefits of quitting at any stage should be emphasised.

Social support and housing

In pregnancy, the prevalence of domestic violence has been shown to be as high as 20% in England.[31] Pregnancy is a time when abuse may start or escalate. More than 30% of cases start during pregnancy.[5,6]

Healthcare professionals need to be alert to the symptoms or signs of domestic violence and women should be given the opportunity to disclose it in an environment where they feel secure. Whenever possible, all women should be seen alone at least once during the antenatal period to enable disclosure more easily if they wish. There should be local strategies for referral to a local multidisciplinary support network to whom the woman could be referred if necessary (Box 4.3).

Work hazards and particular considerations

The majority of women can be reassured that it is safe to continue working during pregnancy. Employers have a statutory obligation to protect the health and safety of new and expectant mothers and are obliged to undertake an individual risk assessment, but there are no clear guidelines regarding the level of risk at which adjustments should be made for pregnant workers. A national guideline exists on physical and shift work.[32]

Box 4.3 Indicators of domestic abuse relevant to maternity care

- Late booking and/or poor or non-attendance at antenatal clinics
- Repeat attendance at antenatal clinics, the GP's surgery or hospital emergency department for minor injuries or trivial or nonexistent complaints
- Unexplained admission
- Noncompliance with treatment regimens or early self-discharge from hospital
- Repeat presentation with depression, anxiety, self-harm and psychosomatic symptoms
- Injuries that are untended and of several different ages, especially to the neck, head, breast, abdomen and genitals
- Sexually transmitted disease and frequent vaginal or urinary tract infections and pelvic pain
- Poor obstetric history
- The constant presence of the partner at examinations, who may be domineering, answer all the questions for her and be unwilling to leave the room
- The woman appears evasive or reluctant to speak or disagree in front of her partner

▇ Training

All clinical staff must undertake regular, written and documented audited training for the identification and initial management of referral for serious medical and mental health conditions that, although unrelated to pregnancy, may affect pregnant women or recently delivered mothers. Basic intermediate and advanced life support skills should be improved.

Maternity service providers and clinical directors must ensure that all clinical staff caring for pregnant women actually learn from any critical events and serious untoward incidents occurring in their trust or practice. Plans for achieving this should be documented at the end of each incident report form.

Staffing and manpower planning

Antenatal care is largely delivered by multidisciplinary teams of midwives and specialist teams. Units must ensure that all the team members are up-to-date with local policies and protocols. Staffing levels in maternity units should conform to the national agreed template.

Every serious untoward incident should be critically reviewed and the lessons learned actively disseminated to all clinical staff, risk managers and administrators. The precise educational actions taken as a result must be recorded, audited and regularly reported to the trust board by the clinical governance lead.

Audit

Each unit should audit its level of adherence to the national quality indicators and the standards of maternity care as agreed by the four Royal Colleges, such as:[33]

- number and percentage of pregnant women with pre-existing medical conditions to whom specialist preconception counselling is offered
- number and percentage of pregnant women at booking who have their body mass index calculated and noted (target 100%)
- number and percentage of staff whose safety and clinical skills training requirements have been identified and addressed in their annual appraisal report (target 100%)
- number and percentage of women counselled and screened for haemoglobinopathies and booked for hospital-based antenatal care.[34]

The provision of courses and a record of attendees should be regularly audited to reinforce, familiarise and update all staff with local procedures, equipment and drugs.

References

1. Department of Health. *Changing Childbirth: Report of the Expert Maternity Group*. London: HMSO; 2003.
2. Singh D, Newburn M, editors. *Access to Maternity Information and Support; the Experiences and Needs of Women Before and After Giving Birth*. London: National Childbirth Trust; 2000.
3. King's Fund. *Safe Births: Everybody's Business. An Independent Inquiry into the*

      Safety of Maternity Services in England. London: King's Fund; 2008 [www.kingsfund.org.uk/publications/safe_births.html].

4. National Institute for Health and Clinical Excellence. *Antenatal Care: Routine Care for the Healthy Pregnant Woman*. NICE Clinical Guideline 62. London: NICE; 2008 [http://guidance.nice.org.uk/CG62].

5. Confidential Enquiry into Maternal and Child Health. *Why Mothers Die 2000–2002. The Sixth Report of the Confidential Enquiries into Maternal Death in the United Kingdom*. London: RCOG Press; 2004.

6. Lewis G, editor. *Saving Mothers' Lives: Reviewing Maternal Deaths to Make Motherhood Safer 2003–2005. The Seventh Report of the Confidential Enquiries into Maternal Deaths in the United Kingdom*. London: CEMACH; 2007 [www.cmace.org.uk/getdoc/319fb647-d2c6-4b47-b6a0-a853a2f4de1b/Maternal-1.aspx].

7. Rowe RE, Garcia J. Social class, ethnicity and attendance for antenatal care in the United Kingdom: a systematic review. *J Public Health Med* 2003;25:113–9.

8. Department of Health. *National Service Framework for Children, Young People and Maternity Services Standard 11: Maternity Services*. London: DH; 2004 [www.dh.gov.uk/en/Publicationsandstatistics/Publications/PublicationsPolicyAndGuidance/Browsable/DH_4094336].

9. Department of Health; Partnerships for Children, Families and Maternity. *Maternity Matters: Choice, Access and Continuity of Care in a Safe Service*. London: DH; 2008 [www.dh.gov.uk/en/Publicationsandstatistics/Publications/PublicationsPolicyAndGuidance/DH_073312].

10. Healthcare for London. *A Framework for Action Pre-report: Maternity and Newborn Clinical Working Group*. London: NHS [www.healthcareforlondon.nhs.uk/a-framework-for-action-2/].

11. HM Government. *PSA Delivery Agreement 19: Ensure Better Care for All*. London: HMSO; 2007 [www.hm-treasury.gov.uk/d/pbr_csr07_psa19.pdf].

12. Timmins CL. The impact of language barriers on the healthcare of Latinos in the United States: a review of the literature and guidelines for practice. *J Midwifery Women's Health* 2002;47:80–96.

13. Healthcare Commission. *Women's Experiences of Maternity Care in the NHS in England: Key Findings from a Survey of NHS Trusts Carried Out in 2007*. London: Commission for Healthcare Audit and Inspection; 2007 [www.cqc.org.uk/publications.cfm?fde_id=7962].

14. Mahmood TA. Obesity and pregnancy: an obstetrician's view. *Br J Diabetes Vascular Disease* 2009;9:19–22.

15. Department of Health. *High Quality Care for All: NHS Next Stage Review Final Report*. London: The Stationery Office; 2008 [www.dh.gov.uk/en/publicationsand-statistics/publications/publicationspolicyandguidance/DH_085825].

16. Department of Health. *Quality Accounts Toolkit: Advisory Guidance for Providers of NHS Services Producing Quality Accounts for the Year 2009/2010*. London: DH; 2010 [www.dh.gov.uk/en/Publicationsandstatistics/Publications/PublicationsPolicy AndGuidance/DH_112359].

17. NHS Information Centre. Indicators for Quality Improvement. 2010 [https://mqi.ic.nhs.uk/].

18. NHS Connecting for Health. Clinical dashboards [www.cfh.nhs. uk/clindash].

19. Royal College of Obstetricians and Gynaecologists. *Maternity Dashboard: Clinical Performance and Governance Scorecard*. Good Practice No. 7. London: RCOG;

2008 [www.rcog.org.uk/womens-health/clinical-guidance/maternity-dashboard-clinical-performance-and-governance-score-card].

20. NHS Screening Programmes. NHS Fetal Anomaly Screening Programme [www.fetalanomaly.screening.nhs.uk].

21. Howarth E, Stimpson L, Barran D, Robinson A. *Safety in Numbers. A Multi-site Evaluation of Independent Domestic Violence Advisor Services*. London: The Henry Smith Charity; 2009 [http://drop.io/safetyinnumbers].

22. Plant MA, Miller P, Plant ML. Trends in drinking, smoking and illicit drug use among 15 and 16 year olds in the United Kingdom (1995–2003). *J Substance Use* 2005;10:331–9.

23. Plant MA, Plant ML. *Binge Britain: Alcohol and the National Response*. Oxford: Oxford University Press; 2006.

24. Plant ML, Plant MA. Heavy drinking by young British women gives cause for concern. *BMJ* 2001;323:1183.

25. Mahmood T, Templeton A, Dhillon C, editors. *Models of Care in Women's Health*. London: RCOG Press; 2009. p. 160.

26. Yost NP, McIntire DD, Wians FH Jr, Ramin SM, Balko JA, Leveno KJ. A randomized, placebo controlled trial of corticosteroids for hypremesis due to pregnancy. *Obstet Gynecol* 2003;102:1250–4.

27. Elbourne D, Richardson M, Chalmers I, Waterhouse I, Holt E. The Newbury Maternity Care Study: a randomized controlled trial to assess a policy of women holding their own obstetric records. *BJOG* 1987;94:612–9.

28. Homer CS, Davis GK, Everitt LS. The introduction of a woman-held record into a hospital antenatal clinic: the bring your own records study. *Aust N Z J Public Health* 1999;39:54–7.

29. Lovell A, Zander LI, James CE, Foot S, Swan AV, Reynolds A. The St Thomas's Hospital maternity case notes study: a randomized controlled trial to assess the effect of giving expectant mothers their own maternity case notes. *Paediatr Perinat Epidemiol* 1987;1:57–66.

30. Royal College of Obstetricians and Gynaecologists. *Female Genital Mutilation and its Management*. Green-top Guideline No. 53. London: RCOG; 2009 [www.rcog.org.uk/female-genital-mutilation-and-its-management-green-top-53].

31. Department of Health. *Responding to Domestic Abuse: a Handbook for Health Professionals*. London: DH; 2005 [www.dh.gov.uk/en/Publicationsandstatistics/Publications/PublicationsPolicyAndGuidance/DH_4126161].

32. Royal College of Physicians of London; NHS Plus. *Physical and Shift Work in Pregnancy: Occupational Aspects of Management. A National Guideline*. London: RCP; 2009 [www.rcplondon.ac.uk/clinical-standards/hwdu/Pages/OHCEU-guidelines.aspx].

33. Royal College of Anaesthetists, Royal College of Midwives, Royal College of Obstetricians and Gynaecologists, Royal College of Paediatrics and Child Health. *Standards for Maternity Care. Report of a Working Party*. London: RCOG Press; 2008 [www.rcog.org.uk/womens-health/clinical-guidance/standards-maternity-care].

34. Department of Health. *Sickle Cell, Thalassemia and Other Haemoglobinopathies*. Report of a Working Party of the Standing Advisory Committee. London: Department of Health; 1999.

CHAPTER 5

Antenatal fetal abnormality screening

Donna Kirwan and Alan Cameron

Key points

✓ From a public health perspective, the identification of anomalies can improve perinatal morbidity and mortality, as conditions may be identified early in pregnancy and managed accordingly.

✓ Specific measures must be taken to become risk averse, as opposed to risk reactive, by conforming to all elements of quality assurance: standards, defining roles and responsibilities, training, qualified and competent staff, audit and monitoring and using approved tools for the job.

▓ Introduction

The UK National Screening Committee, an NHS policy advisory group to the Government, was established in 1996 at the request of the Chief Medical Officer of England to set out a framework for the evaluation and implementation of national screening programmes in the English, Scottish and Welsh National Health Services. The primary aim of the committee is to promote a systematic approach to screening programmes so that they are not introduced into the NHS unless there is robust evidence to support the technology and to advise on the appropriateness of the implementation. The National Screening Committee advises whether or not a screening programme should be started, continued or stopped. So, by bridging the gap between research evidence and policy making, future service standards, audit, quality control and monitoring can become integrated in local NHS services.

To bring conformity at a national level, the UK National Screening Committee integrated different screening programmes into three main domains, each reflecting the stages of the health screening lifecycle. These domains are the Fetal, Maternal and Child Health Group, the Adult Screening and Cancer Screening Programmes. In 2007, ultrasound screening for fetal anomalies and the NHS Down Syndrome Screening Programme were united, since both programmes focus on the identification of anomalies.

■ What women want

The Audit Commission's study, *First Class Delivery: A National Survey of Women's Views of Maternity Care,* highlighted that women were dissatisfied with the amount and quality of information available about antenatal screening procedures.[1] Sixty-nine percent agreed that they received verbal information and 60% received information leaflets, leaving a substantial portion who disagreed or were unsure about what they had been given.

Women's views were also explored in a systematic review of 74 primary studies.[2] Key findings were the need for professionals to be knowledgeable about obstetric scanning and for women to be prepared about the scanning event and the minutiae that practitioners may take for granted. There is no doubt that ultrasound is appealing to women simply because of its visual properties, but the review highlighted that ultrasound also has the potential to amplify maternal anxiety.

Recorded Delivery: A National Survey of Women's Experience of Maternity Care extrapolated views from a random sample of 4800 women selected by the Office for National Statistics.[3] Key findings were that many women were able to access information about Down syndrome screening before 12 weeks of pregnancy, which would provide sufficient time to consider the implications of the screening programme. This is in contrast to some women from black and minority ethnic groups who were not offered or recalled for screening. There was, however, a general paucity of pretest information about the reasons for blood tests and other procedures, which essentially invalidates the consent process.

In the largest maternity report to be commissioned, 45 000 women were invited to participate and over 26 000 responded.[4] Ninety-four percent of women 'who wanted a screening test to check whether their baby was at increased risk of developing Down syndrome, said they had the test', but 88% of women said they had no choice about the test. Similarly, of those who were fortunate to book early (less than 12 weeks of gestation), 60% received a dating scan between 8 and 14 weeks. However, around 10% of women, despite booking before 12 weeks, were not offered a dating scan. Again, 29% felt that they were not given an option to accept or decline the booking scan offer and 27% said the same about the anomaly scan, although they were content with the pretest information given to them.

Key findings emanating from several surveys suggest that communication in its broader sense seemed to be a problem, in that midwives did not offer Down syndrome screening or scanning as 'options' but as a 'routine part of their pregnancy', despite the National Programme's efforts to provide educational materials, tools and training events to promote the concept of informed choice.

■ National guidance and clinical guidelines

Screening is a complex service to deliver; the sometimes contentious issues surrounding the detection of malformation and termination bring with them a number of ethical debates, despite both programmes promoting parental choice. High-quality guidance, specifically policy and programme standards, is therefore a necessity for trusts offering a screening service and, for easy access, all documents are available on the Fetal Anomaly Screening Programme website (http://fetalanomaly.screening.nhs.uk).

The model of best practice for Down syndrome screening makes clear that trusts should be providing a screening test that has a detection rate of 75% or above and a false positive rate of 3% or less.[5] The combined, triple and quadruple tests meet these requirements. Currently, all trusts provide either the triple or quadruple test from 15 weeks and 45% provide combined screening (nuchal translucency and serum) in the first trimester. Recent data collated by the programme centre suggest that this number is due to increase as 63 (41%) primary care trusts come on board by the end of 2010.

Ultrasound is a key component of the combined test requiring sonographers to extend their scope of practice to acquire nuchal translucency imaging skills. With funding from the Department of Health, a national framework has been established to provide continuous quality assurance, training and supervision of qualified practitioners.

◼ Fetal anomaly screening

It is acknowledged that screening for congenital malformations is demanding and time-consuming and it is hoped the new fetal anomaly scan standards that provide minimal and achievable targets will improve ways of working. Trusts must make efforts to apply all the standards to provide a well-controlled programme. However, it is likely that some trusts will be quicker than others. We have therefore described below a few of the standards that trusts should action in the first instance.

Establishment of a coordinating group

All hospital offering obstetric ultrasound should have a trust ultrasound multidisciplinary screening group to oversee the clinical management, governance and quality of the fetal anomaly screening service. Setting up a central communication hub is paramount so that all staff can plan and evaluate what is happening 'at the coalface', monitoring and reporting performance, as well as communicating national policy and developing strategy to cope with any adverse occurrence that may surface unexpectedly. In 2002, just 48% of trusts had a multidisciplinary screening group in place, which is unsatisfactory.

A dynamic multidisciplinary ultrasound team should be central to every trust scan service. Lead individuals will be required for different elements of the screening programme but, overall, the new standards recommend that a lead screening sonographer and deputy be nominated to oversee and coordinate the day-to-day running of the service.

Explicit written arrangements

In ameliorating maternal anxiety and ensuring that the woman receives prompt care and treatment, the new standards recommend that a report of the ultrasound examination should be communicated to the referring clinician within one working day. Additionally, it is also advised that review is undertaken by an obstetric ultrasound specialist within three working days or by a fetal medicine unit within five working days if the woman so wishes. Obviously, the choice of review will be at the discretion of the referrer, depending on pregnancy gestation and the severity of the lesion identified.

Consent

Regrettably, too many women have undergone screening unwittingly, where they might have declined if they had understood the potential implications beforehand. The RCOG and General Medical Council consider consent in the context of a wider process; that is, involving discussion and decision making at each stage of the screening care pathway.[6-8] As such, it is recommended that all women are informed early in pregnancy about screening as 'an option rather than an inevitable aspect of routine antenatal care' and offered information. In meeting the race, diversity and equality agenda, staff should ensure that a professional interpreter is present during the clinical consultation for those women whose first language is not English.

Image capture, storage and archiving

Dramatic improvements in image technology have resulted in efficient ways of archiving and storing ultrasound images and reports for the purposes of providing information for women, evaluating practice through audit and monitoring and holding evidence for legal require- ments. In overstretched clinical services, it is difficult for staff to manually record and store and keep safe hard-copy data. It is imperative that every trust works towards an auditable electronic hospital reporting system to support the fetal anomaly screening service.

■ Down syndrome screening

Historically, Down syndrome screening was offered as a simple blood test from 15 weeks of gestation until the Department of Health policy came into force in April 2003 recommending first-trimester methods.[5] There is much commonality between the Down syndrome screening and Fetal Anomaly Screening Programme standards, in that good screening pro- grammes need a central coordinating group, explicit written arrangements, consent, training and professional competence and monitoring. The national Down Syndrome Screening Quality Assurance Support Service (DQASS) provides an independent audit of laboratory data and statistical support and has made great strides in improving the statistical procedures involved in the production of a patient-specific risk calculation.

Compared with second-trimester screening, combined screening performs better but is generally more demanding on capacity (equipment, time and skill) and quality assurance, owing to the multistepped composition. The Department of Health has allocated funding to establish a national nuchal translucency supervisory, training and quality assurance infrastructure to continue to improve the quality of the combined programme as a whole.

Naturally, there will be some women who will go on to have invasive or diagnostic testing by way of amniocentesis or chorionic villus sampling with associated procedure-related losses. In collaboration with Antenatal Screening Wales, policy, standards and protocols to complement the RCOG Green-top Guidelines have been developed for clinicians with the aim of standardising practice and minimising miscarriage.[9]

Service modelling and care pathways

In understanding the complexities of the woman's journey through the Down syndrome and ultrasound screening system, a number of care pathways have been produced that highlight the main characteristics of each programme where choices can be taken (for example, Figure 5.1).

Special issues related to service delivery

Down syndrome screening

There are many factors that can affect the interpretation of Down syndrome screening and, for this reason, accurate information should be provided, together with the maternal serum sample, to the screening laboratory. Data derived from DQASS have demonstrated significant changes in risk when these details are inaccurate.

The analysis and interpretation of combined screening should be undertaken by the local screening laboratory where staff trained and experienced in Down syndrome screening can generate a risk result using the appropriate equipment.

Women should not be expected to have two scan appointments (dating and nuchal translucency) for combined screening. A single ultrasound appointment should be arranged for the purposes of pregnancy dating, nuchal translucency assessment and blood sampling, which inevitably will reduce costs and save time for both the woman and the trust.

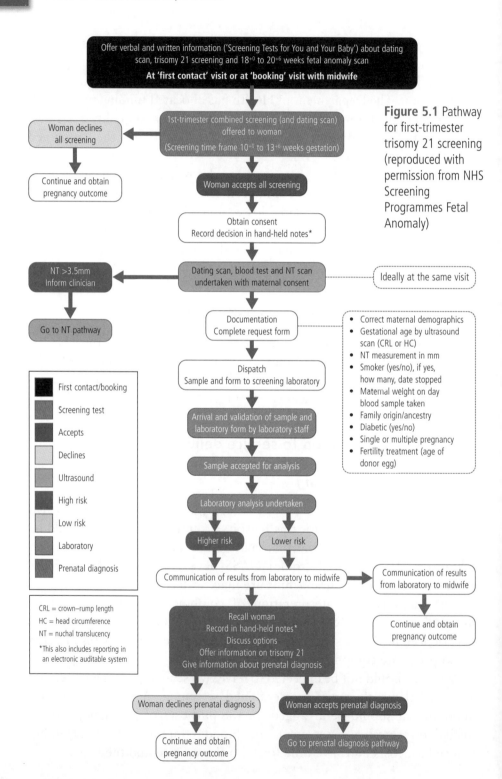

Figure 5.1 Pathway for first-trimester trisomy 21 screening (reproduced with permission from NHS Screening Programmes Fetal Anomaly)

Fetal anomaly screening

Until a few years ago, scanning equipment was purchased directly by hospital trusts from commercially known suppliers. Replacing ultrasound equipment can be expensive. The programme centre recommends that trusts adhere to the NHS supply chain guidance when planning to procure equipment.

As part of quality assurance, CNST and continuing professional development requirements and in line with the NHS Constitution for England, professional development, education and training are considered mandatory. A webpage dedicated to all Fetal Anomaly Screening Programme resources can be sourced at http://fetalanomaly.screening.nhs.uk/educationalresources.

Training

Since the inauguration of the Down syndrome screening standards in 2003, staff have been able to access a succession of education and training resources and events developed by the National Programme Centre in response to requests generated from a national training needs analysis.[10] Two online resources have been tailor-made to support the implementation of combined screening and the national fetal anomaly standards. The first of these, Condensed Education Module for Trisomy 21 (CEM T21), is a compact educational resource constituting approximately 60–90 minutes of web-based learning time that is aimed at sonographers undertaking nuchal translucency scanning.[11] The second initiative is a new web-based interactive resource mapped against the standards and NHS Knowledge and Skills Framework comprising video sequences, 'talking heads' and a resource 'tool-box'.

Staffing and manpower planning

The Society of Radiographers has published a study recommending the action required to increase the number of sonographers, which at the moment accounts for about 200 practitioners.[12] Sickness, repetitive strain injury, retirement and limited student placements are just some examples that have unfortunately reduced the number of practitioners employed within the obstetric ultrasound fraternity. Recommendations include 'increasing the number of trainee sonographers by up to 50%, enabling postgraduate programmes to accept a much wider range of applicants, continue with CASE-accredited [Consortium for the Accreditation of Sonographic Education] postgraduate diplomas and certificates procured by local strategic health authorities, commission short "focused" ultrasound courses and commission direct entry undergraduate programmes, followed by a preceptorship year'.

Audit

Since 2001, a succession of national audits has been undertaken that have proved fruitful in terms of improving services. The extent of the routine examination of the fetal heart serves as a useful example. Recommendations by the RCOG in 2000 stated that 'if resources allow', the cardiac outflow tracts, face and lips 'could be added' to the list of views recommended. Many cardiac anomalies are revealed only if the cardiac outflow tracts are visualised and, as a consequence, the prenatal detection of cardiac anomalies is low. In 2002, trust ultrasound departments were asked to confirm which fetal structures were routinely examined during the ultrasound examination.[13] In 2002, 98% of trusts examined all four chambers of the heart and 57% examined the outflow tracts of the heart. In 2008, the Programme Centre undertook a further audit and reported that 100% of trusts examined the four chambers and 75% examined the outflow tracts,[14] representing an improvement in the screening offered.

Future research

The past 30 years have seen astonishing advances in antenatal screening. The development of serum biochemistry as a means of predicting the risk of Down syndrome has been significant. Developments in the science and art of ultrasound have made it a highly desirable modality that is here to stay until new developments come along.

Research on fetal nucleic acids in maternal plasma is showing promise as a potential way forward to diagnose fetal genetic disorders in the future.[15] A single maternal blood test to analyse cell-free fetal DNA or RNA has benefits in terms of avoiding the 'multistepped' procedures currently in place. As for all National Screening Committee programmes, the technology will need to be meticulously evaluated before endorsing it as a population screening programme.

In utero treatments have for some time been used to treat a number of fetal anomalies or conditions. Intrauterine fetal transfusion for rhesus disease, alloimmune thrombocytopenia and parvovirus infection is established, as is laser ablation therapy for twin-to-twin transfusion. Several fetal medicine services in North America provide fetal surgery for myelomeningocele, a common form of spina bifida. Long-term outcome data are currently being collected by the Management of Myelomeningocele Study and until these are reviewed we can only stay temporarily optimistic about future surgical remedy.[16] Magnetic resonance imaging promises new insights into fetal diagnosis and is a possible way to complement difficult ultrasound diagnoses. However meaningful these interventions are in terms of improving diagnosis, their implementation will require more financial resources and strict criteria for referral.

References

1. Garcia J, Redshaw M, Fitzsimmons B, Keene J. *First Class Delivery: A National Survey of Women's Views of Maternity Care*. London: Belmont Press; 1998.
2. Garcia J, Bricker L, Henderson J, Martin AM, Mugford M, Neilson J, et al. Women's views of pregnancy ultrasound: a systematic review. *Birth* 2002;29:225–50.
3. Redshawe M, Rowe R, Hockley C, Brocklehurst P. *Recorded Delivery: A National Survey of Women's Experience of Maternity Care 2006*. Oxford: National Perinatal Epidemiology Unit, University of Oxford; 2007 [http://www.npeu.ox.ac.uk/recorded-delivery].
4. Healthcare Commission. *Women's Experiences of Maternity Care in the NHS in England: Key Findings from a Survey of NHS Trusts Carried Out in 2007*. London: Commission for Healthcare Audit and Inspection; 2007 [http://www.cqc.org.uk/_db/_documents/Maternity_services_survey_report.pdf].
5. Department of Health. *Model of Best Practice 2003; Down's Syndrome Screening*. London: DH; 2003.
6. Department of Health. *Good Practice in Consent: Achieving the NHS Plan Commitment to Patient-centred Consent Practice*. Health Service Circular 2001/023. London: NHS Executive; 2001.
7. General Medical Council. *Consent Guidance: Patients and Doctors Making Decisions Together*. London: GMC; 2008 [http://www.gmc-uk.org/guidance/ethical_guidance/consent_guidance_index.asp].
8. Royal College of Obstetricians and Gynaecologists. *Obtaining Valid Consent*. Clinical Governance Advice No. 6. London: RCOG; 2008 [http://www.rcog.org.uk/womens-health/clinical-guidance/obtaining-valid-consent].
9. NHS Fetal Anomaly Screening Programme; Antenatal Screening Wales; NHSD Antenatal and Newborn Screening Programme. *Amniocentesis and Chorionic Villus Sampling: Policy, Standards and Protocol*. Exeter: NHS FASP; 2007 [http://fetalanomaly.screening.nhs.uk/standardsandpolicies].
10. Harcombe J. *National Education and Training Needs Analysis for Antenatal Screening and the Newborn Blood Spot Screening Services Across England 2007*. Exeter: NHS Fetal Anomaly Screening Programme; 2007 [http://cpd.screening.nhs.uk/tna].

11. UK National Screening Committee; NHS Fetal Anomaly Screening Programme. CEMT21: Condensed Education Module for Trisomy 21 (Down's syndrome) [http://fetalanomaly.screening.nhs.uk/CEMT21/index.html].

12. Society of Radiographers. *Analysis of Ultrasound Workforce Survey 2009*. London: Society of Radiographers; 2009 [http://doc-lib.sor.org].

13. Whittle M, Honest H. *Antenatal Ultrasound Screening: Ultrasound Survey of England 2002*. Exeter: National Screening Committee; 2005.

14. Maddocks F, Powell H, Day J, Ward P. *Ultrasound Survey of England 2008: Mapping of 1st and 2nd Trimester Fetal Screening Services in the NHS*. Exeter: NHS Fetal Anomaly Screening Programme; 2009 [http://fetalanomaly.screening. nhs.uk/reports].

15. Wright CF, Chitty, LS. Cell-free fetal DNA and RNA in maternal blood: implications for safer antenatal testing. *BMJ* 2009;339:b2451. DOI: 10.1136/bmj.b2451.

16. MOMS: Management of Myelomeningocele Study [www.spinabifidamoms.com].

CHAPTER 6

Antenatal care for low-risk pregnancy

Suzanne Truttero

Key points

✓ Women should be encouraged to book early in their pregnancy.
✓ Antenatal care for women with a current low-risk pregnancy should be provided by a midwife.
✓ Women want to see the same midwife at every antenatal check-up.
✓ Antenatal screening should be offered in accordance with the National Screening Committee recommendations.
✓ Women should be offered information regarding antenatal education.

■ Introduction

The risk status of any pregnancy can change at any point throughout the antenatal period. It is therefore vital that each pregnant woman has an up-to-date plan of care and her risk status is assessed at every contact throughout pregnancy. Antenatal care for women with a low-risk pregnancy is predominately provided by midwives supported by maternity support workers and other professionals. Midwives will make a direct referral to a consultant gynaecologist or obstetrician where a deviation from the normal occurs and a clinical opinion or referral is necessary. Care may also be shared between the midwife and the woman's GP. Where a pre-existing medical condition is identified, the antenatal care will be managed by the appropriate medical team(s) and the midwife will continue to provide midwifery care.

One of the most important aspects of antenatal care is the 'booking' appointment, where the midwife records a history from the expectant parents. Successive triennial reports from the Confidential Enquiries into Maternal Deaths in the United Kingdom have identified that access to antenatal care improves clinical outcome for the mother. *Saving Mothers' Lives* identified ten recommendations, two of which relate to the importance of access to antenatal care.[1]

Women should have had their first full booking visit and hand-held maternity record filled in by 12 completed weeks of pregnancy. In England, this is supported by a Public Service Agreement that requires the NHS to ensure women have had a full assessment of needs, risks and choices by the 12th completed week of pregnancy.[2]

The NHS Operating Framework 2009/2010 requires commissioners of health care (primary care trusts) to increase the percentage of women who have seen a midwife or a maternity healthcare professional for a health and social care assessment of needs, risks and choices by 12 completed weeks of pregnancy.[3] NHS trusts in England are expected to achieve at least 90% coverage by 2010/2011. There are wide variations among primary care trusts, which require innovative ways of engaging with mothers as early in pregnancy as possible. Where a woman is already 12 weeks pregnant or more on contact with maternity services, she should be seen within 2 weeks of referral.

The booking appointment is also an opportunity to discuss with expectant parents lifestyle considerations that may impact on the progress of the pregnancy and provides an opportunity to share information regarding maternity rights and benefits.

One of the important aspects of booking early is the benefits from antenatal screening. During pregnancy, it is important that dating and anomaly scans are performed between 8 and 14 weeks and 18 and 23 weeks of gestation, respectively. In addition to ultrasound examination, blood is taken for routine maternal health screening, the results of which may influence the management of the pregnancy.

What women want

The Healthcare Commission conducted a survey of 26 000 women in relation to their experiences of maternity care in the NHS in England.[4] The key findings were:

- 91% said they first saw a health professional about their pregnancy as soon as they wanted

- 81% of women said they had a choice about where to have their baby, although only 57% said they were given the choice of having their baby at home
- 94% of women who wanted a screening test for Down syndrome said they had the test
- 90% of respondents had the name and telephone number of a midwife they could contact during the pregnancy.
- However, of those respondents who had seen a midwife for their antenatal check-up appointments, 43% had not seen the same midwife and 36% said they were not offered any antenatal classes provided by the NHS.

We are aware that women want high-quality, personal care with greater choice over place of birth, and care provided by a named midwife.[5] This was concluded by a process of the ten strategic health authorities in England each establishing a maternity and newborn group to develop a vision for the pathway of maternity care within their region.

National guidance and clinical guidelines

The National Institute for Health and Clinical Excellence (NICE) published guidance on the routine care of the healthy pregnant woman, outlining a schedule of appointments and the type of screening available.[6] All women should be offered screening for Down syndrome (see chapter 5). Local evidence-based guidelines for the routine care of healthy pregnant women should be informed by the clinical guideline and include information regarding common symptoms of pregnancy.

The antenatal period provides an opportunity to exclude conditions that would require care from professionals in addition to the midwife. The NHS Choices website (www.nhs.uk/Pages/HomePage.aspx) provides access to the Pregnancy Care Planner, where women can obtain information regarding pregnancy and receive information regarding the developing fetus.[7]

The King's Fund report, *Safe Births Everybody's Business*, recommended that 'existing standards should be distilled into a smaller number that are critical to safety'.[8] The Royal Colleges of Obstetricians and Gynaecologists, Midwives, Anaesthetists and Paediatrics and Child Health achieved this in June 2008. They examined 50 publications and identified 800 existing standards, many of which were duplicated, and published *Standards for Maternity Care*, which follows the pathway of maternity care.[7]

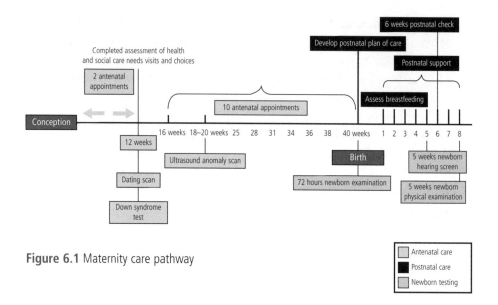

Figure 6.1 Maternity care pathway

Service modelling and care pathways

The pathway above (Figure 6.1) provides details of antenatal care for women with an uncomplicated pregnancy. There are many different models of maternity care that will be influenced by a number of factors. Models of care cannot be considered in isolation as the case mix and available workforce skill mix will impact upon what is available and appropriate for the women being cared for. The Healthcare Commission identified that case loading and team midwifery models of care improved continuity of care and women's satisfaction with the service.[4]

Special issues related to service delivery

It is important that women have direct access to advice by appropriately trained professionals during pregnancy. The establishment of Maternity Direct under the aegis of NHS Direct in certain parts of the country has led to a reduction in antenatal admissions.[9] Providing such a service via a telephone helpline reduces the need for hospital-based maternity care.

Most maternity services have a day assessment unit that provides screening for possible complications of pregnancy and avoids unnecessary hospital admissions. Day assessment units are normally run by midwives and have immediate access to medical staff. This facility can be accessed by any professional providing antenatal care.

Training

Midwives are the specialists of normality and are trained to diagnose pregnancy and assess and monitor women holistically throughout the antenatal period. Midwives are able to provide seamless care and interventions, where appropriate, in partnership with women and other care providers.

Multidisciplinary training should be provided for maternity professionals in relation to domestic abuse. Up-to-date knowledge of the screening tests during pregnancy is required, as recommended by the National Screening Committee and the NICE routine antenatal care guidelines.[6]

Saving Mothers' Lives identified that all clinical staff must undertake the following training:[1]

- the identification and initial management of and referral for serious medical and mental health conditions that, although unrelated to pregnancy, may affect pregnant women
- the early recognition and management of severely ill pregnant women and improvement of basic, immediate and advanced life support skills.

The Clinical Negligence Scheme for Trusts requires maternity services to undertake a training needs analysis of all its staff and prescribes topics for training.[10]

Staffing and manpower planning

There will be many factors that influence the number of staff required and this will be informed by both the case mix of women requiring care and the skill mix of the workforce. The majority of maternity services are using the RCOG Maternity Dashboard, which monitors workforce trends in conjunction with clinical activity and outcomes.[11] This is invaluable for reviewing the capacity of the maternity service. In relation to antenatal care, it will specifically identify the percentage of bookings against the number of births and provide an indication of the reasons for variation.

The National Screening Committee advises that trusts employ a maternity 'test and screening coordinator' to support expectant parents and provide updates on screening for maternity staff.[4]

Audit

Good antenatal care should be viewed as an investment to ensure the mother and baby are in the best possible state of health before the birth. Any audit process of childbirth should include a review of the antenatal care to see if it had any relationship to the birth outcome.

Maternity services should audit the percentage of women who 'booked' by the 12th completed week of pregnancy. More importantly, services should identify those women who booked after 12 completed weeks of pregnancy and the reasons why, to address any barriers to accessing early maternity care.

Audits should be carried out to ascertain how many women recalled seeing the domestic abuse information and whether they understood it, and modifications should be made accordingly.

Figure 6.1 demonstrates the pathway for a low-risk first pregnancy.

References

1. Lewis G, editor. *Saving Mothers' Lives: Reviewing Maternal Deaths to Make Motherhood Safer 2003–2005. The Seventh Report of the Confidential Enquiries into Maternal Deaths in the United Kingdom.* London: CEMACH; 2007 [http://www.cmace.org.uk/getdoc/319fb647-d2c6-4b47-b6a0-a853a2f4de1b/Maternal-1.aspx].
2. HM Government. *PSA Delivery Agreement 19: Ensure Better Care for All.* London: HMSO; 2007 [http://www.hm-treasury.gov.uk/d/pbr_csr07_psa19.pdf].
3. Department of Health. *The Operating Framework for 2009/10 for the NHS in England.* London: DH; 2008 [http://www.dh.gov.uk/en/Publicationsandstatistics/Publications/PublicationsPolicyAndGuidance/DH_091445].
4. Healthcare Commission. *Women's Experiences of Maternity Care in the NHS in England: Key Findings From a Survey of NHS Trusts Carried Out in 2007.* London: Commission for Healthcare Audit and Inspection; 2007 [http://www.cqc.org.uk/publications.cfm?fde_id=7962].
5. Department of Health. *High Quality Care For All: NHS Next Stage Review Final Report.* CM 7432. London; TSO; 2008 [http://www.dh.gov.uk/en/publicationsandstatistics/publications/publicationspolicyandguidance/DH_085825].
6. National Institute for Health and Clinical Excellence. *Antenatal Care: Routine Care for the Healthy Pregnant Woman.* NICE Clinical Guideline 62. London: NICE; 2008 [http://guidance.nice.org.uk/CG62].

7. Royal College of Anaesthetists, Royal College of Midwives, Royal College of Obstetricians and Gynaecologists, Royal College of Paediatrics and Child Health. *Standards for Maternity Care. Report of a Working Party*. London: RCOG Press; 2008 [http://www.rcog.org.uk/womens-health/clinical-guidance/standards-maternity-care].
8. King's Fund. Safe Births: Everybody's Business: An Independent Inquiry into the Safety of Maternity services in England. London: King's Fund; 2008 [http://www.kingsfund.org.uk/publications/safe_births.html].
9. NHS Direct. New maternity services [www.nhsdirect.nhs.uk/article.aspx?name=T3NewMaternityServices].
10. NHS Litigation Authority. Clinical Negligence Scheme for Trusts: Maternity Clinical Risk Management Standards Version 1 2010/11 [http://www.nhsla.com/News/#{A0A8EE5C-A421-4925-AD44-6DF4E3ED8DDC}].
11. Royal College of Obstetricians and Gynaecologists. *Maternity Dashboard: Clinical Performance and Governance Scorecard*. Good Practice No 7. London: RCOG; 2008 [http://www.rcog.org.uk/womens-health/clinical-guidance/maternity-dashboard-clinical-performance-and-governance-score-card].

CHAPTER 7

Antenatal care for women with pre-existing medical, obstetric or mental health conditions

Jessica Moore and Baskaran Thilaganathan

Key points

✓ Local trusts and perinatal network teams should develop guidelines for the identification and provision of further support to women identified as high risk during pregnancy.

✓ A referral care pathway should be in place so that women are referred to high-risk clinics.

✓ A multidisciplinary team should be in place to provide care to women with previously known medical condition(s), according to agreed care plans.

✓ A fast-track care pathway should be in place within regional maternity networks for early referral to a specialist team for assessment.

✓ A care pathway should be in place in each region for routine and emergency situations in high-risk pregnancies.

✓ Perinatal networks should ensure that robust communication plans are in place between all professionals and the woman.

■ Introduction

Women with pre-existing medical and obstetric problems are at increased risk of complications in pregnancy. Such high-risk pregnancies result in increased maternal, fetal and neonatal morbidity and mortality. It is well recognised that the impact of psychological morbidity in the perinatal period on the woman and her family is significant and often underestimated by carers. Unidentified or inadequately treated mental illness during pregnancy has serious consequences postnatally, such as self-harm or suicide. One of the main aims of antenatal care is to identify pre-existing risk factors early to ensure optimum management of the pregnancy by the relevant multiprofessional teams in the most appropriate environment (Figure 7.1).

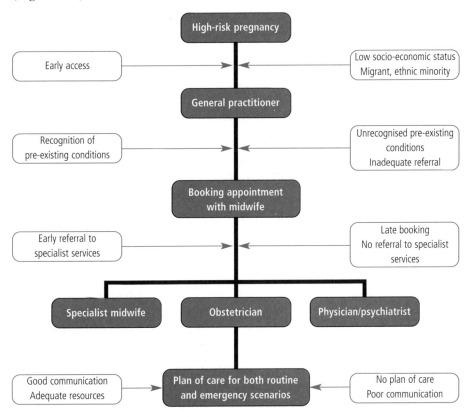

Figure 7.1 Identifying risk factors for pre-existing conditions

What women want

Maternity Matters describes a comprehensive programme for improving choice, access and continuity of care for pregnant women.[1] It sets out a strategy to put women and their families at the centre of local maternity services provision. The document stresses that all women must have informed choice over the type of care they receive. In women with high-risk pregnancies complicated by pre-existing conditions, the plan of care should involve at least the hospital consultant obstetrician, a named or specialist midwife and may also involve specialist physicians.

National surveys of women's views about their antenatal care have demonstrated that the majority of women thought that they received a high standard of care but, in a significant proportion of cases (30–60%), the women considered that they did not have informed choice about the delivery of health care and place of birth.[2,3] It is apparent that women with a high-risk pregnancy would have a narrower range of healthcare choices. However, it is apparent that this does not preclude the need for providing information about the appropriate choices to such women.

■ National guidance and clinical guidelines

In 2008, the National Institute for Health and Clinical Excellence (NICE) issued guidelines for routine antenatal care of healthy pregnant women.[4] However, these guidelines stress that women suffering from pre-existing medical problems are outside their scope. Such pre-existing medical or mental health issues should be highlighted in the GP's referral letter to maternity services. This highlights the role of the GP, who is the only healthcare professional to have full access to a woman's complete medical history.

The NICE routine antenatal care guideline states that women should have access to maternity services at 8–10 weeks to allow them time to plan for their pregnancy effectively. Specific recommendations from the 2003–2005 Confidential Enquiries into Maternal Deaths in the United Kingdom (CEMD) advise GPs to 'fast track' referrals to appropriate physicians if women have serious medical conditions such as epilepsy.[5] The advice further states that GPs should not rely on conventional referral pathways to the obstetrician or midwife as these may introduce delays that compromise the woman's care. The most commonly referred conditions include epilepsy, diabetes and cardiac disease. Common medical conditions that confer a higher risk to the pregnancy but are often unrecognised at referral are obesity and mental health disorders.

The RCOG published *Standards for Maternity Care* in June 2008 to help develop national standards for maternity care.[6] They recommend that staff working with women in the antenatal period should be competent at recognising, advising and referring women who would benefit from more specialist services. This usually involves an obstetrician trained in maternal medicine at a local or regional level. Other specialists may also be involved, including physicians, perinatal psychiatrists and anaesthetists. It is also important, where possible, to promote normality and this is often best supported by regular midwifery involvement. Continuity of care by the same midwife throughout the pregnancy will provide the best support and advocacy for a woman with a high-risk pregnancy. As with any care provided by a multidisciplinary team, communication between team members is essential to optimise care.

▓ Service modelling and care pathways

Maternity Matters stresses the need for clear protocols on when, how and where to refer women for more specialist care. The pattern of antenatal care can vary considerably depending on the local geography and resources. Most frequently, obstetricians with a maternal medicine interest will run a joint service with specialist physicians. Typically, women will be seen in a joint clinic, but it is not unusual for them to be seen in sequential clinics, especially when the prevalence of the medical disorder does not justify setting up a regular joint clinic. An alternative model of care is for the specialist clinic to be run by an obstetric physician who is a general physician rather than a specialist in a particular field. The former model allows women to have continuity of care by the most appropriate specialist for their particular medical disorder before, during and after the pregnancy. The advantage of the latter model is that most women can be seen in a single medical clinic without the need to attend multiple specialist clinics in the pregnancy.

Whatever the model of care, there is a need to have protocols and care pathways that are tailored for the local resources. These will need to be updated on a regular basis in line with changes in service provision and emerging evidence and guidelines. Given the multiprofessional nature of the service provision, it is recommended that regular multidisciplinary team meetings be held to review management plans for women with high-risk pregnancies.

Most commonly, the schedule of care is outlined in an integrated care pathway. An integrated care pathway is a multidisciplinary outline of anticipated care, placed in an appropriate timeframe, to help a patient with a specific condition or set of symptoms move progressively through a clinical experience to positive outcomes. Integrated care pathways can also be used as tools to incorporate local and national guidelines into everyday practice, manage clinical risk and meet the requirements of clinical governance.

Special issues related to service delivery

The 2003–2005 CEMD report highlighted the lack of multidisciplinary care for women with pregnancies complicated by existing or new medical or psychiatric problems. Although there has been a growth in the number of multidisciplinary clinics for the most common conditions such as epilepsy, diabetes and cardiac disease, it is clear that some of the women who died did not receive optimum care. In addition, deaths from underlying neurological conditions were highlighted as an area needing increased care in the form of combined neurology or general medical/ obstetric clinics.

Although a large proportion of women were managed in multidisciplinary clinics, they did not always have a clear management plan. Such a plan would include management in emergency situations and details of any additional services required for their care. In short, poor communication has been highlighted as a major shortfall in the care of women with high-risk pregnancies. This includes poor or nonexistent teamworking, inappropriate or too short telephone consultations, a lack of sharing of relevant information between health professionals and poor interpersonal skills.

There are many reasons for and opportunities in the patient care pathway for poor communication to result in substandard care. In terms of access to specialist services, it is apparent that migrant and ethnic minority populations have been identified as groups of women at risk of late referral and undiagnosed existing medical conditions, such as rheumatic heart disease. The clinician should ensure that a comprehensive booking history is taken and a full clinical assessment is made, including a cardiovascular examination. Telephone consultations are increasingly used by the medical and midwifery professions as a means of assessing patients, without appropriate training.

Cardiac disease and mental health in pregnancy were the most common causes of maternal deaths in the 2003–2005 CEMD report. Myocardial infarction was the most common cardiac cause, prompting a low threshold for investigating pregnant women with cardiac symptoms to be recommended. NICE has published guidelines on the provision of antenatal and postnatal mental health.[7] The key recommendation is a proactive enquiry about past and current mental health problems and status. Women who are identified as being at risk of developing serious postnatal mental illness must be assessed by a perinatal psychiatrist to ensure a clear written plan of management for their postnatal care.

Training

In keeping with advice from the Centre for Maternal and Child Enquiries, all medical and midwifery practitioners, particularly specialists in acute medical care, require knowledge of the way that common medical conditions interact with pregnancy. Training programmes for midwives, obstetricians, GPs and psychiatrists should include perinatal psychiatric disorders.

Specialty training in obstetrics and gynaecology includes modular training in maternal medicine for all trainees, with an optional Advanced Training Skills Module (ATSM) for senior trainees who wish to develop and provide expertise in caring for pregnant women with pre-existing medical disorders.[8]

Staffing and manpower planning

There is recognition that women with more complex needs such as those with pre-existing medical problems will require care from more experienced obstetricians. The role of regional centres is important for the provision of fetal and maternal medical care for more complex pregnancies.

Maternity Matters addresses the issue that the shorter working week imposed by the 48-hour Working Time Regulations will bring more difficulties for trainees and consultant obstetricians to obtain and maintain their skills to an appropriately high standard. Not all hospitals can provide a full range of specialist obstetrics services. Overcoming this problem may require not only reconfiguration of services but also the development of cross-site working practices. The needs of the local population must be taken into account when planning a service in terms of providing the correct care, particularly in areas where there are large numbers of women from migrant and ethnic minority populations.

The RCOG report *The Future Workforce in Obstetrics and Gynaecology* addresses the needs of the workforce within obstetrics and gynaecology.[9] Currently, there are approximately 5–10 subspecialty trained and 10–15 maternal medicine ATSM trained Certificate of Completion of

Training holders qualifying each year. By contrast, there are approximately 200 maternity units nationally, which all require either consultant subspecialists or consultants with a special interest. This apparent discrepancy would need to be addressed to optimise the staff-to-patient ratio.

The Birthrate Plus survey provides a detailed staffing profile of midwifery and non-midwifery establishments for all areas of service based on current and projected activity and models of care.[10] This survey is biased towards the intrapartum case mix, as this has a major impact on the hospital workload and the midwifery establishment. The provision of a robust antenatal service to women with high-risk pregnancies does not require a significant increase in midwifery numbers but rather the appointment of a few specialist caseload midwives to provide a point-of-care contact for the mother, to maintain a sense of normality for her and to help communication between the specialists.

Audit

Standards for Maternity Care states that documentary evidence of at least the following should be available:[6]

- multidisciplinary joint clinics (joint diabetes/antenatal care)
- percentage of women with a pre-existing medical condition who are assessed by a consultant obstetrician
- percentage of women with a pre-existing medical condition who are seen by an appropriate multidisciplinary team
- percentage of women who have a documented plan of care
- local joint working arrangements with a perinatal mental health network
- percentage of staff trained in mental health issues.

The use of well designed integrated care pathways should allow not only delivery of a robust service but also the simultaneous collection of the required audit data.

Future research

Areas for future research include:

- evidence- and governance-based integrated care pathway templates for specialist services

- reasons for late referral from general practice to specialist services
- communication between both different points of care (medical clinics, delivery suite and so on) and professionals.

References

1. Department of Health. *Maternity Matters: Choice, Access and Continuity of Care in a Safe Service*. London: DH; 2008 [http://www.dh.gov.uk/en/Publicationsand statistics/Publications/PublicationsPolicyAndGuidance/DH_073312].
2. Hundley V, Rennie AM, Fitzmaurice A, Graham W, van Teijlingen E, Penney G. A national survey of women's views of their maternity care in Scotland. *Midwifery* 2000;16:303–13.
3. Redshawe M, Rowe R, Hockley C, Brocklehurst P. *Recorded Delivery: A National Survey of Women's Experience of Maternity Care 2006*. Oxford: National Perinatal Epidemiology Unit, University of Oxford; 2007 [http://www.npeu.ox.ac.uk/recorded-delivery].
4. National Institute for Health and Clinical Excellence. *Antenatal Care: Routine Care for the Healthy Pregnant Woman*. NICE Clinical Guideline 62. London: NICE; 2008 [http://guidance.nice.org.uk/CG62].
5. Lewis G, editor. *Saving Mothers' Lives: Reviewing Maternal Deaths to Make Motherhood Safer 2003–2005. The Seventh Report of the Confidential Enquiries into Maternal Deaths in the United Kingdom*. London: CEMACH; 2007 [http://www.cmace.org.uk/getdoc/319fb647-d2c6-4b47-b6a0-a853a2f4de1b/Maternal-1.aspx].
6. Royal College of Anaesthetists, Royal College of Midwives, Royal College of Obstetricians and Gynaecologists, Royal College of Paediatrics and Child Health. *Standards for Maternity Care. Report of a Working Party*. London: RCOG Press; 2008 [http://www.rcog.org.uk/womens-health/clinical-guidance/standards-maternity-care].
7. National Institute for Health and Clinical Excellence. *Antenatal and Postnatal Mental Health: Clinical Management and Service Guidance*. NICE Clinical Guideline 45. London: NICE; 2007 [http://guidance.nice.org.uk/CG45].
8. Royal College of Obstetricians and Gynaecologists. ATSM: Maternal Medicine [http://www.rcog.org.uk/curriculum-module/atsm-maternal-medicine].
9. Royal College of Obstetricians and Gynaecologists. *The Future Workforce in Obstetrics and Gynaecology England and Wales: Full Report*. London: RCOG; 2009 [http://www.rcog.org.uk/files/rcog-corp/uploaded-files/RCOGFuture WorkforceFull.pdf].
10. Birthrate Plus. *Ratios for Midwifery Workforce Planning At National, SHA and Local Level*. Nottingham: Birthrate Plus; 2009 [http://www.birthrateplus.co.uk].

CHAPTER 8

Antenatal care for women developing medical or obstetric problems during pregnancy

Roshni Patel and Philip Owen

Key points

✓ The majority of women experience no complications during pregnancy, but a significant proportion requires additional multidisciplinary care to maximise healthy outcomes.

✓ The provision of written patient information will aid in the understanding of conditions about which women may have no prior knowledge.

✓ Recognised referral pathways must be established and accessible.

✓ Care of women developing complications must adhere to locally adapted national evidence-based guidelines where such guidelines exist.

✓ Regular participation in multidisciplinary training is an essential component of maintaining staff expertise and familiarity.

✓ Well-constructed and completed audit cycles will highlight deficiencies in service provision and stimulate efforts to raise standards.

■ Introduction

Each woman hopes that her pregnancy will be free of complication, but medical and obstetric complications are common in the antenatal period and, even if they are minor, they can be a source of anxiety to the pregnant woman and her family. During the antenatal period conditions unique to pregnancy may develop, such as pre-eclampsia, gestational diabetes mellitus and obstetric cholestasis, in addition to the less commonly encountered new pathologies, whether medical, surgical or mental. The obstetrician and midwife will invariably feel more comfortable with those conditions that are pregnancy-related, but women may still benefit from the expertise of other specialties and referral to tertiary level units if the conditions are severe.

Where concurrent illnesses not directly related to pregnancy are encountered, obstetricians and midwives will need more support and, here, close contact with other specialists is essential. Pregnancy often affects the interpretation of and limits the applicability of certain investigations and treatments such that continued obstetric input remains appropriate when the woman's principal specialist is not regularly caring for pregnant women.

What women want

To support women through what is potentially a difficult time, providing high-quality information is essential. Expectant mothers require information about the effects of the condition on themselves and their unborn child. This information may be available through a variety of media but, as a minimum, patient leaflets should be available, presented in a range of languages as appropriate to the local population. In the case of less frequently encountered conditions, women should be directed to recognised support groups and recommended online information. It is essential that women are provided with balanced information that is representative of local care pathways.

One of the best methods of supporting women and placing the management plan within the context of local practice is contact with specialist midwives. These midwives will be able to provide continuity of care and act as the woman's advocate. Specialist midwives should be available when women develop gestational diabetes and, where possible, pregnancy-induced hypertension and pre-eclampsia.

National guidance and clinical guidelines

There are several evidence-based guidelines available to assist the clinical management of conditions arising in pregnancy. These include guidelines published by the RCOG (www.rcog.org.uk/guidelines), which include pregnancy-related conditions, such as obstetric cholestasis,[1] and those not associated with pregnancy but with potentially serious complications for mother and fetus, such as chickenpox in pregnancy.[2] These guidelines provide peer-reviewed advice on clinical management and include information on the level of evidence for all statements. The guidelines are reviewed at regular intervals and thus provide the latest evidence-based information. The majority of these guidelines are accompanied by a relevant patient information leaflet, which can be accessed using the guidelines web link. The National Institute for Health and Clinical Excellence (www.nice.org.uk) and the Scottish Intercollegiate Guidelines Network (www.sign.org.uk) also provide evidence-based guidelines relating to pregnancy and childbirth.

Maternity units will already have local guidelines for the management of women developing common conditions, such as pre-eclampsia, gestational diabetes and obstetric cholestasis, and such locally adapted guidelines require regular updating. Units that do not have such guidelines must create relevant guidance reflecting national recommendations, adapted to suit local needs and resources.

The development of a modified obstetric early warning system will assist with the timely diagnosis of critical illness and will help to ensure prompt referral to other specialists and the transfer of women to high-dependency and intensive care units.

Service modelling and care pathways

All obstetricians need to be aware of the management of women developing medical and obstetric problems during pregnancy. All women developing these problems need access to a consultant obstetrician for assessment and subsequent consultant-led care if required. The transfer of antenatal care from midwifery-led care to shared or consultant care must follow clear pathways and must be easily achieved by community midwives, GPs and other hospital-based specialists, thus avoiding delays in diagnosis and treatment.

Each maternity unit should have a clinician with an interest and expertise in the care of high-risk pregnancies. This lead clinician should, together with colleagues from within obstetrics and other specialties, generate local protocols for the antenatal care of women with high-risk pregnancies. A physician with an interest in maternal medicine is well placed to act as liaison between the departments of obstetrics and medicine and, if the department is of sufficient size, to contribute or lead an obstetric medicine clinic. Where women develop medical complications not related to pregnancy, referral to or consultation with the lead of the local obstetric medicine service is recommended. Combined obstetric and diabetes clinics are well established and a diagnosis of gestational diabetes is a clear indication for referral to such a multidisciplinary service. In conjunction with this, the role of specialist midwives should be developed to enhance the care of women developing medical and obstetric problems. Such midwives play an invaluable role in the coordination of care through their participation in specialist clinics and through their own independent practice.

In the event of acute serious medical conditions, such as pulmonary embolus, pathways need to be clear so that prompt treatment can be started. In such conditions, there should be clear escalation pathways, with the involvement of a senior obstetrician at the earliest stages. Such involvement facilitates communication with other senior specialists (such as radiologists, anaesthetists and neonatologists) for further investigations and planning care, including management in labour. The consultant on-call should be informed of the admission of all sick women admitted with medical or obstetric problems and must be available to review them if necessary.

Women who develop subacute medical or obstetric problems in pregnancy can frequently be appropriately managed in the day assessment setting. An experienced obstetrician should be available to provide advice for these cases. The use of a day assessment unit allows midwifery-led patient care and longer-term follow-up to be arranged. This care pathway has the additional benefit of not unnecessarily occupying inpatient beds. Pregnant women generally prefer to remain as outpatients where possible. However, hospital protocols for common conditions such as pregnancy hypertension and pre-eclampsia require explicit criteria to indicate where outpatient management is no longer appropriate and hospital admission is necessary.

Pregnant women admitted to the accident and emergency department should have their cases discussed with obstetric or midwifery staff unless their complaint is very minor. Ideally, the woman should be reviewed by obstetric and/or midwifery staff before discharge from hospital. Even in the case of minor medical problems, women should be advised to see their community midwife following discharge to ensure continued care and the provision of any follow-up arrangements.

■ Special issues related to service delivery

Maternity service providers need to provide consultant-led care in a setting with adequate facilities with availability of other specialists nearby. Small or geographically remote maternity units may not have access to these facilities and they should have clear referral pathways to other units. This may be for high-risk obstetric facilities and delivery, anaesthesia expertise in an intensive-care setting or access to neonatal intensive care, or all of these. Consideration must be given to the provision of readily available transport for pregnant women requiring transfer following an accepted pattern of referral between the referring and accepting maternity units. It is important to recognise that women developing certain obstetric conditions such as pre-eclampsia may experience a rapid deterioration in their condition that is notoriously difficult to predict.

Following delivery, every effort should be made to keep the mother and her newborn baby in the same unit and return to their base unit should be prioritised once their medical condition allows.

Providers of maternity services must consider women from minority ethnic groups, who may need access to translated written information and professional translators. Women with medical or obstetric problems and concurrent social difficulties should have specific arrangements made for them including access to a named midwife for the duration of their pregnancy, together with involvement of the department of social work.

■ Training

Optimal patient care requires a continuous cycle of training aimed at all components of the multidisciplinary team. Each unit will have a lead clinician for high-risk pregnancies and an RCOG tutor who is responsible for organising local postgraduate educational activities. Together with the lead midwife, these clinicians should ensure that training is provided and should monitor attendance patterns for all staff disciplines. The lead clinician should liaise with clinicians from other specialties to coordinate training and should ideally develop joint training days. Where appropriate, the use of simulated scenarios should be integrated into training days to optimise the understanding of care pathways, particularly for acute illnesses or complications such as severe pre-eclampsia and eclampsia.

Training courses should be repeated at least annually, with interim updates provided in light of major new clinical findings. In addition, training needs to be integrated into staff inductions so that they can be familiarised with local protocols upon commencing a post in a new location. Specific training by way of maternal medicine and advanced antenatal care Advanced Training Skills Modules (ATSMs) are a component of training for many senior obstetric specialty trainees. The curriculum is set by the RCOG and the training is overseen by the local deanery specialty training committee. Theoretical courses relevant to medical complications in obstetrics are provided by the RCOG and others; attendance at such a course is mandatory before completion of the relevant ATSM.

■ Staffing and manpower planning

Complications developing during pregnancy are common. Most illnesses are mild, requiring understanding, surveillance, explanation and timed delivery at term. However, a small number of women will develop more complex disorders requiring considerable staff input of time and expertise. These latter cases are by their very nature unpredictable and become an additional staffing requirement beyond that which is required to provide the routine antenatal and intrapartum service. This must be borne in mind when calculating the number of midwives required per shift so that there is sufficient midwifery staffing available to care for the majority of women at low risk when additional midwifery time is being devoted to these complicated cases.

Training obstetricians to become leads in high-risk obstetrics or maternal medicine involves completion of the appropriate ATSM or subspecialty training. The provision of these training opportunities can be tailored to anticipated forthcoming consultant vacancies such that there is a degree of succession planning and service development.

■ Audit

Regular audit is necessary to ensure that national and local standards of care are being met and if there are shortfalls in practice to address the deficiencies by way of education and expansion or reallocation of resources. Subjects for audit should be decided at a senior level on a regular basis and this is often coordinated by regional audit committees.

Auditing practice against evidence-based national guideline recommendations is appropriate. Dissemination of results should also be considered at a regional or national level, through meetings and publications, if the findings are considered to have wider implications.

■ Future research

There are numerous aspects of antenatal care that require further research and allow focus on specific conditions to reduce morbidity and mortality for mothers and babies. In addition to new research projects, consideration should be given to the use of local patient databases for epidemiological analyses. This form of research is cost-effective and easily translated to patient care.

■ References

1. Royal College of Obstetricians and Gynaecologists. Green-top Guideline No. 43. *Obstetric Cholestasis*. London: RCOG; 2006 [http://www.rcog.org.uk/womens-health/clinical-guidance/obstetric-cholestasis-green-top-43].
2. Royal College of Obstetricians and Gynaecologists. Green-top Guideline No. 13. *Chickenpox in Pregnancy*. London: RCOG; 2007 [http://www.rcog.org.uk/womens-health/clinical-guidance/chickenpox-pregnancy-green-top-13].

CHAPTER 9

Managing risk in antenatal care

Helen Scholefield and Walaá Al-Safi

Key points

✓ Managing risk in antenatal care is dependent on identification of risk factors through risk assessment. Women may move between low and high risk at different stages and risk management processes must ensure that they receive the level of care they need in an effective and safe manner. Such processes need to take into account the multiple settings and providers involved in antenatal care.

✓ Significant risk issues include increasing obesity, pre-existing medical conditions, increasing maternal age, not speaking English, women who do not access care and vulnerable groups.

✓ Risk management should include:
  ○ organisational culture
  ○ risk assessment
  ○ training
  ○ induction
  ○ guidelines
  ○ communication
  ○ audit
  ○ learning from adverse incidents, claims and complaints.

Introduction

Excellent maternity care is comprehensive and flexible enough to respond to the clinical and social needs of women and their families. In recent years, standards of care in maternity services have been investigated and subsequently highlighted in several audits and surveys. Managing risk in antenatal care is dependent upon the identification of risk factors through clinical risk assessment during pregnancy to identify the care that is appropriate to individual women's needs. The National Service Framework sets out the need for flexible services that can respond appropriately to those who may require highly specialised care for existing medical problems, social circumstances and any complications that may develop.[1] Women may move between low- and high-risk categories during pregnancy; risk management processes need to ensure that they receive the level of care they need in an effective and safe manner.

What women want

Most women regard pregnancy as a natural physiological process. Surveys have shown that pregnant women anticipate having as normal a pregnancy and birth as possible. Reports of the maternity and newborn clinical working groups indicate a clear message that women want high-quality, personal care with greater choice over place of birth and care provided by a named midwife.[2] Their ultimate expectation is to exercise choice around how and where they have their child.

The King's Fund has published a study of women's views of safety in maternity care.[3] This found that older, better-educated women tended to be more assertive and to expect a greater share in decision-making. However, this was not always the case and many women who had started by wanting to make the decisions were quite happy to hand over control when problems developed. Women often referred to childbirth as being a natural process but many accepted that childbirth carries inherent risks. There were indications that cultural differences could alter a woman's perception of safety. Wider, more systemic safety issues were also mentioned throughout the course of the interviews, from the reputation of certain hospitals to adherence to safety protocols. In some instances, women found that strict adherence to hospital policies led to an inflexible and untailored approach to individual care. It was noted that the nature of childbirth means that certain safety concerns may have come to light only in retrospect. Even when concerns were raised, an ultimately happy outcome still made women reluctant to describe their overall care as unsafe.

The Healthcare Commission survey of women's experiences of maternity care in the NHS in England found that most women wanted to see a health professional as soon as they wanted, and to have choice and continuity of care and access to antenatal classes.[4]

National guidance and clinical guidelines

These are systematically developed statements used to assist practitioner and patient decisions about appropriate health care for specific clinical circumstances and can improve quality of care by supplying the knowledge practitioners need to put evidence-based medicine into practice. Guidelines are only helpful if they are effectively implemented. Evaluation of their effectiveness through audit and adverse event reporting is important. All guidelines need to be reviewed at regular intervals to incorporate new evidence and issues identified through audit and adverse event reporting.[5]

There is a plethora of national guidance documents on antenatal care including recommendations and guidance from sources such as the Centre for Maternal and Child Enquiries, the National Institute for Health and Clinical Excellence (NICE) and other professional bodies. These are recognised standards against which care is judged and it is important that all units carefully consider how they are implemented, which requires them to be adapted to local needs.[5] To help providers and commissioners negotiate their way through them, the report of a working party on standards for maternity care pulled the salient points of all these together into one document and provided guidance for the development and audit of equitable, high-quality services across the UK.[6]

NICE guidelines and interventional procedures guidance provide evidence-based information for use by clinicians and pregnant women to make decisions about appropriate treatment in specific circumstances. Those relevant to antenatal care are shown in Box 9.1. The RCOG has a menu of evidence-based Green-top Guidelines (www.rcog.org.uk/guidelines) and other guidelines are also available from the Scottish Intercollegiate Guidelines Network (www.sign.org.uk).

Service modelling/care pathways

Maternity Matters describes a comprehensive programme for improving choice, access and continuity of care, setting out a strategy that will put women and their partners at the centre of their local maternity service provision.[7] The key aim is to improve the quality of service, safety,

Box 9.1 NICE guidance on antenatal care

Antenatal Care: Routine Care for the Healthy Pregnant Woman
NICE Clinical Guideline CG62. March 2008
[http://guidance.nice.org.uk/CG62]

Caesarean Section
NICE Clinical Guideline CG13. April 2004
[http://guidance.nice.org.uk/CG13]
Discusses issues about the information women can expect to receive
about caesarean section as well as the benefits and risks of having a
caesarean birth compared with a vaginal birth

**Diabetes in Pregnancy: Management of Diabetes and its
Complications From Pre-Conception to the Postnatal Period**
NICE Clinical Guideline CG63. March 2008
[http://guidance.nice.org.uk/CG63]

**Antenatal and Postnatal Mental Health: Clinical Management
and Service Guidance**
NICE Clinical Guideline CG45. February 2007
[http://guidance.nicc.org.uk/CG45]
Underlines the importance of recognising mental health problems
during pregnancy and in the first year after giving birth

Percutaneous Fetal Balloon Valvuloplasty for Aortic Stenosis
NICE Interventional Procedure Guidance IPG175. May 2006
[http://guidance.nice.org.uk/IPG175]

**Percutaneous Fetal Balloon Valvuloplasty for Pulmonary Atresia
with Intact Ventricular Septum**
NICE Interventional Procedure Guidance IPG176. May 2006
[http://guidance.nice.org.uk/IPG176]

Percutaneous Laser Therapy for Fetal Tumours
NICE Interventional Procedure Guidance IPG180. June 2006
[http://guidance.nice.org.uk/IPG180]

Insertion of Pleuro-Amniotic Shunt for Fetal Pleural Effusion
NICE Interventional Procedure Guidance IPG190. September 2006
[http://guidance.nice.org.uk/IPG190]

Box 9.1 NICE guidance on antenatal care (continued)

Therapeutic Amnioinfusion for Oligohydramnios During Pregnancy (Excluding Labour)
NICE Interventional Procedure Guidance IPG192. November 2006
[http://guidance.nice.org.uk/IPG192]

Intrauterine Laser Ablation of Placental Vessels for the Treatment of Twin-to-Twin Transfusion Syndrome
NICE Interventional Procedure Guidance IPG198. December 2006
[http://guidance.nice.org.uk/IPG198]

Septostomy With or Without Amnioreduction for the Treatment of Twin-to-Twin Transfusion Syndrome
NICE Interventional Procedure Guidance IPG199. December 2006
[http://guidance.nice.org.uk/IPG199]

Fetal Vesico-Amniotic Shunt for Lower Urinary Tract Outflow Obstruction
NICE Interventional Procedure Guidance IPG202. December 2006
[http://guidance.nice.org.uk/IPG202]

Fetal Cystoscopy for Diagnosis and Treatment of Lower Urinary Outflow Outflow Tract Obstruction
NICE Interventional Procedure Guidance IPG205. January 2007
[http://guidance.nice.org.uk/IPG205]

Guidance under development:
Pregnancy and Complex Social Factors
Clinical Guideline. Publication date: September 2010
[http://guidance.nice.org.uk/CG/Wave14/29]

Hypertensive Disorders During Pregnancy
Clinical Guideline. Publication date to be confirmed
[http://guidance.nice.org.uk/CG/Wave15/10]

Multiple Pregnancy
Clinical Guideline. Publication date: September 2011
[http://guidance.nice.org.uk/CG/Wave16/8]

outcomes and satisfaction for all women through offering informed choice around the type of care that they receive and improved access to services, while ensuring continuity of care and support. The aim of pregnancy care pathways is to ensure that there are clear pathways in place to address the needs of pregnant women with various health problems during pregnancy, intrapartum and postnatally in accordance with national guidelines. These care pathways are likely to impact positively on pregnant women to ensure that their health needs are identified in a timely way and appropriate referrals/interventions/care planning put in place.

Maternity Matters recommends the use of the 'antenatal assessment tool' to identify pregnant women for whom additional care is necessary. It also underlines the role of good communication between healthcare professionals and women, as well as the use of written information tailored to the woman's needs. At the first contact with a healthcare professional, each pregnant woman is assessed by the antenatal assessment tool to identify risk factors and plan antenatal care accordingly. She is offered information on various health issues, antenatal screening, the anomaly scan as well as risks and benefits of the screening tests. At booking (ideally by 10 weeks), further information on fetal development and pregnancy requirements is offered. This approach aims to identify women who may require additional care for medical or social reasons. Pregnant women are then grouped into low-risk (midwifery-only care) and increased-risk (midwifery and obstetric care) categories, with the potential to identify a third group of women who are particularly vulnerable and at increased risk of maternal and perinatal death.

All women should receive the NICE pathway of antenatal care with additional requirements being 'bolted on' to this.[8] The pathway of care should be monitored in a way that ensures compliance with guidance for antenatal, intrapartum mental health and postnatal care.[4]

■ Special issues related to service delivery

Antenatal care is provided in multiple settings that pose different challenges compared with intrapartum care, where risk is more overt. It is vital to ensure that same governance structures are in place across these. A Confidential Enquiries into Maternal and Child Health report has highlighted a number of risk issues including obesity, pre-existing medical conditions, increasing maternal age, non-English-speaking women who do not access care and vulnerable groups, all of which need to be considered in the delivery of an antenatal care service.[9]

Effective interaction between different agencies is essential, including communication among primary, secondary and tertiary care, social services and mental health services. It is vital that adequate communication occurs between all of these services. All relevant professionals must be kept informed of the plan of care and any complications. Adequate discharge information is essential.

In addition to verbal communication, documentation helps those looking after the woman to be aware of what has been planned or done. Documentation should include any discussions that have taken place with the woman and the relevant management plan. Good communication skills are one of the most important aspects of patient care;[5] it is often on these that our patients judge the care they receive. Recognising women's expectations is important; they are likely to be dissatisfied with their care and complain if their expectations are not met. For non-English-speaking women, access to interpreters is necessary and trusts need to have a robust policy in place for this.

Patient information is another key area. This can be by providing either adequate verbal explanation or written information and other formats such as Braille and audio tapes. Information may need to be provided in different languages. Patient information leaflets are extremely useful but must not be used as a replacement for adequate explanation and discussion.

Training

Training and induction of staff are essential elements in providing safe and effective care in the antenatal period, as unfamiliarity with the task increases the risk of error 17-fold and inexperience four-fold.[5] Training programmes must be integrated with the local induction process whereby staff members are informed of the risk management principles and all associated policies. Such programmes need to cover the specific requirements of the diverse settings of antenatal care such as the different community settings, hospital antenatal clinics, maternal and fetal medicine and antenatal day assessment. The generic requirements of all staff must be identified. Training matrices are useful in identifying what training is essential for every level of staff. It is also important to tailor training needs to individuals.

The following areas are particularly important in managing risk in ante-natal care and should be included in induction and be regularly updated:

- screening: to ensure that staff members have the necessary knowledge and competencies to implement local and national screening programmes
- supervised practice: this allows staff to develop their skills and competencies to be assessed while minimising the risk to patients, and is particularly relevant in the use of ultrasound and invasive procedures
- equipment: matrices are useful in identifying which members of staff need training on particular items of equipment, limiting their use to those appropriately trained
- risk management: local procedures and guidelines, systems in place in the organisation for patient safety and incident reporting. It is important to stress the systems approach to give staff the confidence to report adverse events.

Staffing and manpower planning

Shortage of time increases the risk of error ten-fold.[5] High-quality maternity services rely on having an appropriate workforce with the leadership, skill mix, competencies and well defined roles and responsi-bilities to provide excellent care at the point of delivery.[6] Service providers should ensure that the staff mix provides multidisciplinary teams with agreed shared objectives.[4]

Where geographically relevant, commissioners and providers should ensure that staffing levels and competencies on labour wards comply with the standards of Clinical Negligence Scheme for Trusts, Standards in Maternity Care.[6,10] The staffing profile should reflect that of the local population to ensure strengthened services for women from disadvant-aged and minority groups.[6] All healthcare professionals directly involved in childbirth should be trained to carry out neonatal and adult life support. Women with medical problems such as diabetes, epilepsy and mental health disorders should be cared for by a team of specialist midwives and/or obstetricians. This applies to women with additional needs such as teenagers, asylum seekers or those with disabilities or substance misuse.[6] Every pregnant woman should have a designated midwife from the point of diagnosing pregnancy.

There should be a lead consultant obstetric anaesthetist with responsibility for the organisation and management of the specialist anaesthetic service within consultant-led units. All women requiring regional or general anaesthesia should be seen and assessed by an anaesthetist before an elective procedure.[6]

■ Future research

There is a dearth of research into risk management in antenatal care. NICE has recognised several areas of particular importance:

- The antenatal assessment tool: multicentre validation studies are required in the UK to evaluate the use of the antenatal assessment tool in identifying women who:
  - can remain within or return to the routine antenatal pathway of care
  - may need additional obstetric care for medical reasons
  - may need social support and/or medical care for a variety of socially complex reasons.
- Information for pregnant women: alternative ways of helping healthcare professionals to support pregnant women in making informed decisions should be investigated.
- Fetal growth and wellbeing: prospective research is required to evaluate the diagnostic value and effectiveness of predicting small-for-gestational-age babies.

■ References

1. Department for Education and Skills; Department of Health. *National Service Framework for Children, Young People and Maternity Services. Maternity Services. Standard 11.* London: Department of Health; 2004 [http://www.dh.gov.uk/en/ Publicationsandstatistics/Publications/PublicationsPolicyAndGuidance/Browsable/ DH_4094336].
2. Department of Health. *High Quality Care for All: NHS Next Stage Review Final Report.* London: TSO; 2008 [http://www.dh.gov.uk/en/Publicationsandstatistics/ Publications/PublicationsPolicyAndGuidance/DH_085825].
3. Magee H, Askham J. *Women's Views about Safety in Maternity Care: A Qualitative Study.* London: King's Fund; 2008 [http://www.kingsfund.org.uk/ current_projects/maternity_services_inquiry/index.html].
4. Healthcare Commission. *Women's Experiences of Maternity Care in the NHS in England: Key Findings From a Survey of NHS Trusts Carried Out in 2007.* Commission for Healthcare Audit and Inspection [http://www.cqc.org.uk/_db/_ documents/Maternity_services_survey_report.pdf].

5. Scholefield H. Risk management in obstetrics. *Curr Obstet Gynaecol* 2005; 15:237–43.

6. Royal College of Anaesthetists, Royal College of Midwives, Royal College of Obstetricians and Gynaecologists, Royal College of Paediatrics and Child Health. *Standards for Maternity Care. Report of a Working Party*. London: RCOG Press; 2008 [http://www.rcog.org.uk/womens-health/clinical-guidance/standards-maternity-care].

7. Department of Health. *Maternity Matters: Choice, Access and Continuity of Care in a Safe Service*. London: DH; 2008 [http://www.dh.gov.uk/en/Publicationsand statistics/Publications/PublicationsPolicyAndGuidance/DH_073312].

8. Department of Health. Better Care: Better Lives. Improving outcomes and experiences for children, young people and their families living with life-limiting and life-threatening conditions. London: DH; 2008 [http://www.dh.gov.uk/en/Publicationsandstatistics/Publications/PublicationsPolicyAndGuidance/DH_083106].

9. Confidential Enquiry into Maternal and Child Health. *Perinatal Mortality 2005: England, Wales and Northern Ireland*. CEMACH: London; 2007 [http://www.cmace.org.uk/publications/CEMACH-publications/Maternal-and-Perinatal-Health.aspx].

10. NHS Litigation Authority. Clinical Negligence Scheme for Trusts: Maternity Clinical Risk Management Standards Version 1 2010/11 [http://www.nhsla.com/News/#{A0A8EE5C-A421-4925-AD44-6DF4E3ED8DDC}].

CHAPTER 10

Intrapartum care for women assessed as low risk in labour

Mervi Jokinen

Key points

- ✓ Wherever the birth takes place, the principles and practice will remain the same, but organisational and service infrastructures should be in place to support delivery of midwifery-led care for women assessed to be at 'low risk' in labour.
- ✓ Local information of care pathways that have been developed with active contribution of women will increase confidence and ownership in accessing maternity care.
- ✓ A woman with a healthy pregnancy and spontaneous onset of labour should be afforded care that maintains this status.
- ✓ Teaching and training needs to emphasise the importance of recognising normal physiological progress of labour to avoid unnecessary medical interventions.

■ Introduction

More women are entering into labour naturally. Most of these women are assessed as 'low risk' at the start of the labour and should receive midwifery-led care as recommended by current government policies and clinical guidelines.[1,2] Midwifery-led care is considered to be care offered to women with uncomplicated pregnancies in which midwives take primary professional responsibility for care. Such care may be provided at home, in birth centres or in obstetric units. Currently, the majority of births in the UK take place in obstetric units. As a result of service mergers, establishing new neonatal networks and current policy drivers in the NHS, an increase in the number of birth centres and a potential increase in the number of home births is anticipated. This chapter explores how policies, current standards and practices can be integrated to improve women's access and promote confidence and trust in the services provided as well as having a maternity workforce who use resources effectively.

Wherever the birth takes place, principles and practice will remain the same. However, organisational and service infrastructures have to be in place to support delivery of midwifery-led care.[3-5] For safety and quality of care, protocols and care pathways are recommended, but midwives and obstetricians need to remember that each woman's care is individual and her journey through the labour is dynamic.[6]

The challenges raised by labelling women as being at 'low risk' or 'high risk' should not be based on professional rivalries or fears but on ensuring that a woman receives the care she needs.

What women want

The White Paper *Our Health, Our Care, Our Say* emphasises that listening to users and engaging them in developing values and philosophy is crucial for service delivery.[7] In turn, this should be the driver for the expectations in commissioning of services.[8,9] An understanding of short- and long-term health benefits from maintaining principles of low-risk labour care should be an economic driver as much as the more immediate cost of normal birth.

Two reports looking at women's experiences of care in labour highlighted important issues such as feeling in control in a physical environment that supports mobility and comfort in labour.[10,11] Being left alone in a labour ward was associated with an increased need for pharmacological pain management.

It is vital to hear what women want. Using women's focus groups and complaints pathways can provide much useful information. Locally developed care pathways with active contribution from women will increase confidence and ownership in accessing maternity care.

Commissioners have to undertake an assessment of local childbearing population needs to ensure that the services they buy provide choice and optimum care for all women. They should monitor local maternity service delivery by requesting audit data on choice of place of birth, facilities provided, numbers of spontaneous vaginal births, one-to-one care in labour and women's experiences.

National guidance and clinical guidelines

Evidence-based normal midwifery care is the integration of best evidence with clinical expertise and user values. The Royal College of Midwives (RCM) has produced a set of evidence-based guidelines for midwifery-led care in labour to support midwives' practice and reduce unnecessary intervention. These guidelines can be found on the RCM website (www.rcm.org.uk/college/standards-and-practice/practice-guidelines).

The National Institute for Health and Clinical Excellence(NICE) *Intrapartum Care* guideline recognises the elementary pathway for healthy women and babies in labour receiving midwifery-led care.[2]

The professionals agree that each organisation should have locally agreed clinical guidelines for midwifery-led labour care for low-risk women. External organisations involved with assessments in the safety and quality of care (Clinical Negligence Scheme for Trusts, CNST; Care Quality Commission) require the same information. These should address not just clinical care but also referral criteria and transfers from low-risk to high-risk care. Maximising the outcomes of labour care for low-risk women must acknowledge a smooth transition from midwifery-led to team-based care if so required.

Service modelling and care pathways

Maternity Matters has set out a framework for recommended service models.[1] The Welsh Assembly All Wales Clinical Pathway for Normal labour[12] and Scottish Pathways for Maternity Care are also relevant.[13] The care pathway that a woman follows cannot be divided into isolated episodes. The advantage of setting the pathway parameters is that the woman should receive optimum care at whatever stage of the journey she is at and a continuous assessment is made upon her progress through that pathway.

A linked principle we should set is that a woman with a healthy pregnancy and spontaneous onset of labour should be afforded care that maintains this status. In labour care, this means that service modelling takes into account early labour/latent phase, active labour and immediate post-birth care. It needs to plan carefully where and how this care is provided and aim for continuity of care.

It is recognised that 'activities' in early labour can impact on the physiology of labour. NICE has a definition of latent phase and there is an agreement that the labour ward may not be the ideal environment during this stage of labour.[2,9,13] The latent phase can be a painful and anxious time for a woman, especially in first pregnancy, confirming or eliminating any expectations of her labour. In addition, the first labour is crucial in setting precedence to other pregnancies. For women, the key aspect is the environment: does it induce confidence and relaxation in the knowledge that labour or birth is not going to be imminent? Some units have set an area for triage care for women in early labour and they have the option of either returning home or going into the antenatal area. The aim is to validate that healthy pregnancy has progressed spontaneously into early onset of labour without any deviation from normal, an action plan discussed with the woman and support offered as required. This is reflected in the first of the 'Ten Top Tips' in the RCM Campaign for normal birth:[9]

'Wait and See

The one single practice most likely to help a woman have normal birth is patience. But in order to be able to let natural physiology take its own time, we have to be very confident in our own knowledge and experience. To do this, we need to be able to acquire more knowledge and experience of normal birth – and know when the time is right to take action.'

In active labour, nationally agreed pathways and guidance set the framework. A sound knowledge of physiology and the mechanism of labour are essential, but practitioners must link this with listening to the woman.

'Listen to her

Women themselves are the best source of information about what they need. However, a medicalised culture of 'knowing best' (where the deferential 'patient' is examined mutely) means that we are not good at asking her. We are also losing our skills in being able to read her non-verbal signals: her body language, gesture, expression, noises and so on. What we need to do is to get to know her, listen to her, understand her, talk to her and think about how we are contributing to her sense of achievement.'

Special issues related to service delivery

Many units and organisations at strategic health authority level have taken on board the self-improvement toolkit by the NHS Institute for Innovation and Improvement.[14] This toolkit encourages the whole organisation and maternity team to self-assess their service delivery by acknowledging the wider determinants (than clinical care) that influence optimal outcome. After studying and looking at top performing trusts they published top ten characteristics in supporting normal birth. The first five are:

- We focus on keeping pregnancy and birth normal.
- We are a real team: we understand and respect roles and expertise.
- Our leaders are visible and vocal.
- Our guidelines are evidence-based and up to date.
- We all practise to the same guidelines: no opting out.

When organisations are self-assessing it is apparent that the quality and value of service delivery are as much dependent on shared values, attitudes, culture and leadership as on clinical guidelines, which also have to reflect team-wide ownership. Poor teamwork is a theme impacting adversely on the outcomes, safety and quality agenda.[2,15] We may perceive that low-risk labour care involves minimal numbers of staff, but the need for close proximity in working with the team will always impact on actions and the level of interventions used. One way to overcome this is to focus on the need of the woman; for example, some women complain about the number of people entering the room.

The decades 1990–2010 have seen a gradual increase in built-in birthing pools in different birth environments. In birth centres, pools are blended into the physical environment of each room and subsequently greater numbers of women give birth in the pool. More commonly, bringing in costly technology such as central electronic fetal monitoring stations is acceptable, as it often fits a team's ethos of labour care. Service planning has to support both low-risk and high-risk labour care pathways with equity.

Training

In line with national maternity standards,[3,16,17] 'skills and drills' programmes in obstetric emergencies are accepted as improving the safety of labour care. The report does not, however, discuss what skills are required in improving the safety of low-risk labour care by maintaining the mother's low-risk status.

Nonmedical interventions facilitating labour are skills that fit easily in a birth centre or home birth environment but can be less evident or topical in a busy obstetric unit. However, they should not be viewed as something that comes naturally to all midwives during preregistration training. Current midwifery education may present few opportunities for student midwives or medical students to observe physiological labour. This, in itself, is an indicator that we are failing to provide appropriate labour care for low-risk women. Providing mandatory training is challenging owing to staff time and financial restrictions, but sessions on water birth, non-pharmacological pain relief strategies, using equipment such as a birthing ball and different positions, are important.

■ Staffing and manpower planning

There is universal agreement that one-to-one care by a midwife for a woman in active labour is requisite. It is an important baseline and does not depend on the risk status of the woman or environment but underpins the level of care required for clinical observations, progress assessments, clinical decision making and psychological and social support. The RCM has produced guidance on staffing levels,[4] which were stated in the *Safer Childbirth* document,[3] giving the recommended ratios for the labour environment.

The CNST has set auditing of these ratios as one of their standard criteria. For low-risk labours, the midwife may be assisted by a maternity care support worker for nonclinical activities. Any birth environment should have a monitoring tool for staffing levels. It should assess the skill-mix and case categories in real time to numbers of midwives.

Current recommendations are for each provider to assess their local population needs and build a care model or structure that facilitates these local needs.[4] The breakout is to design models of care around the needs of women and not those of the organisation. If future maternity services provide diversity of labour environments, strategic manpower planning cannot be sustained on acute and community workforce planning.

Audit

There are many sources recommending audits on labour care and outcomes: RCM birth centre standards,[5] *Safer Childbirth,*[3] *Standards for Maternity Care.*[16] There must be some universal auditing to allow for data comparison nationally or globally, although the aim of auditing must be seen as part of the audit cycle in improving care.

Future research

Previous research in pregnancy and childbirth has focused heavily upon medical and therapeutic interventions and there is a growing interest in increasing research and audit in the area of socio-physiological elements of care for women and their babies. There is a need for a holistic and rounded approach to research and evidence-based practice to contribute to providing care for women, their families and the professional staff providing that care. Effective audit in the range of environments can contribute to a more realistic picture of maternity care and to a balanced examination of outcomes.

References

1. Department of Health. *Maternity Matters: Choice, Access and Continuity of Care in a Safe Service.* London: DH; 2008 [http://www.dh.gov.uk/en/Publicationsand statistics/Publications/PublicationsPolicyAndGuidance/DH_073312].
2. National Institute for Health and Clinical Excellence. *Intrapartum Care: Management and Delivery of Care to Women in Labour.* Clinical Guideline 55. London: NICE; 2007 [http://guidance.nice.org.uk/CG55].
3. Royal College of Obstetricians and Gynaecologists, Royal College of Anaesthetists, Royal College of Midwives and Royal College of Paediatrics and Child Health. *Safer Childbirth: Minimum Standards for the Organisation and Delivery of Care in Labour.* London; RCOG Press; 2007 [http://www.rcog.org.uk/womens-health/clinical-guidance/safer-childbirth-minimum-standards-organisation-and-delivery-care-la].
4. Royal College of Midwives. *Staffing Standard in Midwifery Services.* Guidance Paper No. 7. London: RCM; 2009 [http://www.rcm.org.uk/college/standards-and-practice/guidance-papers].
5. Royal College of Midwives. Standards for Birth Centres in England: A Standards Document. London: RCM Trust; 2009.
6. Department of Health. *National Service Framework for Children, Young People and Maternity Services Standard 11: Maternity Services.* London: DH; 2004 [www.dh.gov.uk/en/Publicationsandstatistics/Publications/PublicationsPolicyAnd Guidance/Browsable/DH_4094336].

7.   Department of Health. *Our Health, Our Care, Our Say: A New Direction for Community Services*. London: HMSO; 2006 [http://www.dh.gov.uk/en/Publications andstatistics/Publications/PublicationsPolicyAndGuidance/DH_4127453].

8.   Healthcare for London. *A Framework for Action*. 2nd ed. London: NHS; 2007 [http://www.healthcareforlondon.nhs.uk/a-framework-for-action-2].

9.   Royal College of Midwives. The RCM Launches 10 Top Tips for a Normal Birth for Midwives and Mothers [http://www.rcm.org.uk/college/media-centre/press-releases/the-rcm-launches-10-top-tips-for-a-normal-birth-for-midwives-and-mothers].

10. Healthcare Commission. *Women's Experiences of Maternity Care in the NHS in England: Key Findings From a Survey of NHS Trusts Carried Out in 2007*. Commission for Healthcare Audit and Inspection [http://www.cqc.org.uk/_db/_documents/Maternity_services_survey_report.pdf].

11. Redshawe M, Rowe R, Hockley C, Brocklehurst P. *Recorded Delivery: A National Survey of Women's Experience of Maternity Care 2006*. Oxford: National Perinatal Epidemiology Unit, University of Oxford; 2007 [http://www.npeu.ox.ac.uk/recorded-delivery].

12. Hunter B. The All Wales Clinical Pathway for Normal Labour: What Are the Experiences of Midwives, Doctors, Managers and Mothers? Final Project Report: A Policy Ethnography to Explore the Implementation of The All Wales Clinical Pathway for Normal Labour. Swansea: Institute of Health Research, School of Health Science, Swansea University; 2007 [http://www.swpho.nhs.uk/resource/item.aspx?RID=72057].

13. NHS Quality Improvement Scotland. *Pathways for Maternity Care*. Edinburgh: NHS QIS; 2009 [http://www.nhshealthquality.org/nhsqis/5989.html].

14. NHS Institute for Innovation and Improvement. *Pathways to Success: a self improvement toolkit- focus on normal birth and reducing caesarean section rates*. NHS Institute for Innovation and Improvement; 2007 [http://www.institute.nhs.uk].

15. King's Fund. *Safe Births: Everybody's Business: An Independent Inquiry into the Safety of Maternity services in England*. London: King's Fund; 2008 [http://www.kingsfund.org.uk/publications/safe_births.html].

16. Royal College of Anaesthetists, Royal College of Midwives, Royal College of Obstetricians and Gynaecologists, Royal College of Paediatrics and Child Health. *Standards for Maternity Care. Report of a Working Party*. London: RCOG Press; 2008 [http://www.rcog.org.uk/womens-health/clinical-guidance/standards-maternity-care].

17. NHS Litigation Authority. Clinical Negligence Scheme for Trusts: Maternity Clinical Risk Management Standards Version 1 2010/11 [http://www.nhsla.com/News/#{A0A8EE5C-A421-4925-AD44-6DF4E3ED8DDC}].

Further reading

Nursing and Midwifery Council. *Midwives Rules and Standards*. London: NMC; 2004 [http://www.nmc-uk.org/Educators/Standards-for-education/Midwives-rules-and-standards/].

Stewart M, McCandlish R, Henderson J, Brocklehurst P. *Review of evidence about clinical, psychosocial and economic outcomes for women with straightforward pregnancies who plan to give birth in a midwife-led birth centre, and outcomes for their babies*. Oxford: National Perinatal Epidemiology Unit; 2005 [http://www.npeu.ox.ac.uk/birthcentrereview].

Williams FL, Florey CV, Ogston SA, Patel NB, Howie PW, Tindall VR. UK study of intrapartum care for low risk primigravidas: a survey of interventions. *J Epidemiol Community Health* 1998;52:494–500.

CHAPTER 11

Intrapartum care for high-risk pregnancies

Sailesh Kumar

Key points

✓ Risk assessment of the woman and fetus prior to labour is essential.
✓ High-risk pregnancies should be delivered in a tertiary centre where multidisciplinary expertise is available.
✓ The views of women and healthcare providers should be taken into account when service development is contemplated.
✓ Compliance with national and RCOG guidelines is essential from both a best practice and a medico-legal perspective.
✓ Further research into intrapartum fetal monitoring and the impact of obstetric interventions on long-term outcomes is needed.

▓ Introduction

Although the vast majority of pregnancies proceed without complications and result in a healthy newborn, others may be more complex because of antenatal or intrapartum conditions. Both pre-existing chronic conditions (hypertension, diabetes mellitus, renal disease and autoimmune disorders) and conditions that arise during pregnancy itself (pre-eclampsia, fetal growth restriction, congenital malformations and multiple pregnancy) can jeopardise the wellbeing of both mother and baby (Tables 11.1 and 11.2). Fetal growth restriction arising from placental insufficiency is a significant cause of perinatal mortality (stillbirth or neonatal death) and morbidity. In addition to perinatal mortality, intrapartum hypoxia, regardless of aetiology, can also cause long-term physical and mental disability (cerebral palsy).

Table 11.1 Medical disorders associated with increased intrapartum risk (modified from the NICE Intrapartum Care guideline, June 2008)[11]

Disease	Medical condition
Cardiovascular	Congenital or acquired cardiac disease Hypertension
Respiratory	Moderate or severe asthma Cystic fibrosis
Haematological	Haemoglobinopathies Red cell alloimmunisation Any maternal or fetal bleeding disorder (e.g. ITP, FAIT/NAIT) Thromboembolic disease
Infective	HIV Tuberculosis
Immune	Systemic lupus erythematosus Scleroderma
Endocrine	Thyroid or adrenal disease Diabetes
Renal	Chronic renal disease Renal transplant
Gastrointestinal	Chronic liver disease Liver transplant
Neurological	Myasthenia gravis Epilepsy Any cerebrovascular disease
Psychiatric	Any disorder requiring inpatient care

Although the majority of fetal neurological injuries predate labour, the intrapartum period is a time of risk of asphyxia and asphyxia-related morbidity and mortality. The extent to which intrapartum asphyxia can be prevented by improved care is controversial, but several investigations and malpractice claims analyses suggest that a significant proportion is preventable.[1-5]

The major contributors to fetal mortality worldwide are obstructed labour and its sequelae (trauma, asphyxia and infection), maternal infections such as syphilis and malaria, birth asphyxia associated with maternal and fetal complications including poor placentation, placental abruption, severe pre-eclampsia and eclampsia, maternal/fetal malnutrition, congenital malformations and umbilical cord complications.[6] There may be variations in the contributions of these different causes between different geographical areas but, in general, these are the major causes of fetal mortality and morbidity.

Table 11.2 Obstetric factors associated with increased intrapartum risk (modified from the NICE Intrapartum Care guideline, June 2008)[11]

Risk	Obstetric factor
Previous obstetric complications	Intrapartum death, stillbirth or neonatal death Neonatal encephalopathy Severe pre-eclampsia Placental abruption with adverse outcome Eclampsia Uterine rupture Massive postpartum haemorrhage Retained placenta requiring manual removal in theatre Caesarean section Shoulder dystocia
Current pregnancy	Multiple birth Placenta praevia Pre-eclampsia or pregnancy-induced hypertension Preterm labour or preterm prelabour rupture of membranes Placental abruption Severe anaemia Confirmed intrauterine death Substance misuse Alcohol dependency requiring assessment or treatment Gestational diabetes Malpresentation Maternal obesity (body mass index >35 kg/m^2) Recurrent antepartum haemorrhage Grand multiparity Increased maternal age
Fetal complications	Fetal growth restriction Fetal macrosomia Abnormal fetal heart rate/Doppler studies Severe oligo/polyhydramnios
Previous gynaecological history	Myomectomy Hysterotomy

Normal intrapartum care

All women, regardless of whether their pregnancies are high or low risk, should be treated with respect and should be in control of and involved in what is happening to them in labour. To facilitate this, it is essential that all healthcare professionals should not only establish a rapport with the woman but also be aware of her expectations for labour. This information should be used to support and guide the woman throughout labour within the constraints of the underlying reason that categorised her pregnancy as high risk in the first place.

Prior to labour, all women should be risk assessed and stratified using either local or national criteria (Tables 11.1 and 11.2). Once this has been done, a judgement needs to be made regarding the mode of delivery. For some conditions the decision is obvious (for instance, placenta praevia), while for others (cardiac disease) it may be equivocal. It is critical that, where appropriate, this judgement is discussed in a multidisciplinary forum and that any decision is made by a senior clinician and carefully documented in the notes. The decision to allow a woman with a high-risk pregnancy a trial of labour must be made before labour with full involvement of the woman in the decision making process. Although there is considerable flexibility for the woman at low risk in many aspects of her care, particularly intrapartum management, this will not apply to a high-risk pregnancy. Clearly, a woman with pre-eclampsia, cardiac disease or fetal growth restriction would be unsuitable for delivery outside a high-risk unit and would require additional monitoring in labour. Many of these pregnancies may be best delivered by elective caesarean section, for either maternal or fetal reasons.

Labour is a dynamic process and, because of this, all healthcare providers should be cognisant of the possibility that, on occasion, even an apparently low-risk pregnancy can suddenly develop intrapartum complications that result in it becoming high risk. In some studies, up to 30% of previously low-risk pregnancies developed complications during labour. Therefore, intrapartum care clinical guidelines should be explicit in reflecting this to ensure that women in this situation then receive increased medical, anaesthesia and midwifery input during labour when appropriate.

Perinatal mortality

In the 2009 report into perinatal mortality in the UK, teenage mothers (aged less than 20 years at delivery) had the highest neonatal mortality rate (4.4/1000 live births) compared with other maternal age groups. In this report, teenage pregnancies contributed 9.6% to overall neonatal mortality in England, Wales and Northern Ireland.[7] It is speculated that this may be because of a number of factors such as social deprivation and a higher rate of preterm delivery in this age group. Extremes of maternal age, non-white ethnicity and maternal social deprivation also continue to be risk factors for stillbirth and neonatal death. In addition, maternal obesity is also likely to be associated with these adverse outcomes.

A study from 2009[8] suggested that suboptimal intrapartum care occurred in 40–50% of cases where there was metabolic acidosis at birth. Most cases of suboptimal care consisted of injudicious use of oxytocin and a failure to act on an abnormal fetal heart rate trace. The authors noted that in many cases there appeared to be a gap between knowledge and clinical practice and that availability of clinical intrapartum guidelines did not reduce the incidence of adverse outcomes. This trend is also supported by various national surveys in the UK suggesting that suboptimal care is responsible for almost 70% of intrapartum fetal deaths.[9–11]

Maternal mortality

Maternal deaths are extremely rare in the UK. In 2003–2005,[12] 149 women died from an obstetric-related cause in the UK, giving a maternal death rate of 7/100 000 maternities. The most common cause of direct death was thromboembolism. Intrapartum causes of maternal mortality are extremely rare; nevertheless, good intrapartum care and monitoring of the woman with a high-risk pregnancy is essential in ensuring a good maternal and fetal outcome. Crucially, this involves identifying the high risk before the onset of labour and instituting appropriate management in labour.

National guidance and clinical guidelines

In the UK, the National Institute for Health and Clinical Excellence (NICE) has published comprehensive guidelines on the intrapartum care of the woman at low risk at term (over 37 weeks of gestation).[11] The guidelines emphasise the importance of continuous clinical governance monitoring and recommend the following:

- Multidisciplinary clinical governance structures (such as a labour ward forum) should be in place to enable the oversight of all places of birth. These structures should include, as a minimum, midwifery, obstetric, anaesthesia and neonatal expertise, and adequately supported user representation.
- In all places of birth, risk assessment in the antenatal period and during labour should be subject to continuous audit.
- Monthly figures of numbers of women booked for, being admitted to, being transferred from and giving birth in each place of birth should be audited. This should include maternal and neonatal outcomes.
- The clinical governance group should be responsible for detailed root-cause analysis of any serious maternal or neonatal adverse outcomes (for example, intrapartum-related perinatal death or seizures in the neonatal period) and consider any 'near misses' identified through risk-management systems.
- The Confidential Enquiry into Maternal and Child Health (CEMACH)[12] and the National Patient Safety Agency (NPSA) *Seven Steps to Patient Safety* document[13] provide a framework for meeting clinical governance and risk-management targets.
- Data must be submitted to the national registries for either intrapartum-related perinatal mortality or neonatal encephalopathy once these are in existence.

In addition, the RCOG recommends that any obstetric service delivery organisation has a robust and transparent clinical governance framework that is applicable to each birth setting.[14] Within this setting, effective multidisciplinary care and good communication should be key factors for good practice. Furthermore, adequate staffing levels of all clinical and support staff are required and these must be reviewed and audited annually. Clinical leadership in promoting good practice and coordinating care is vital. Protocols based on clinical, organisational and system needs should also be available. Professional staff should have the opportunity and support for continuing professional development, including agreed mandatory education and training sessions. Audit of relevant outcomes with attention to any changes or trends is also mandatory.

The factors detailed above are relevant to any clinical setting but are particularly important in an organisation where more women with high-risk pregnancies are cared for.

The other important publication is *Standards for Maternity Care*.[15]

Staffing, manpower planning and training

All maternity units and labour wards should have a lead named midwife, obstetrician, paediatrician and anaesthetist. It is imperative that staffing levels and competencies of staff on labour wards comply with national standards. In the UK, the Clinical Negligence Scheme for Trusts (CNST) or equivalent (Welsh Risk Pool or Clinical Negligence and Other Risk Indemnity Scheme) requires the attainment of certain standards, in terms of both labour ward consultant cover and staff attendance at mandatory education and training days, to ensure compliance with CNST requirements and before a higher level is awarded. A higher level is associated with considerable financial savings to the trust. In addition, consultant obstetric units require a 24-hour anaesthesia and analgesia service with consultant supervision, an adult high-dependency unit and access to intensive care, haematology and blood transfusion. An integrated obstetric, anaesthetic and neonatal care service is vital in providing good intrapartum care to the high-risk woman.

Planning for future manpower requirements is tricky at the best of times. The birth rate in the UK is rising at the present time, fuelled in part by immigration. Many other developed countries have falling or static birth rates and the converse is true for developing countries. What is clear is that obstetric outcomes are better when you have well-staffed units with well-trained staff using clear protocols and guidelines. In the UK, the relevant Royal Colleges recommend between 1.2 and 1.4 whole-time equivalent midwives to one woman for a moderate- to high-risk case mix.[14] The RCOG has also recommended that labour wards supporting large numbers of births (over 5000 a year) and/or a complex case load should be moving towards a 168-hour consultant-based service by 2010.[16] The background to this recommendation is the recognition that the level of activity on the labour ward varies very little during a 24-hour period and that senior presence is therefore required for the totality of the working day, to support and train junior staff and to ensure high-level decision making. This level of cover (midwifery and medical) has major implications for staff in terms of job plans, remuneration and facilities at work, appropriate time off duty as well as work–life balance. The majority of obstetric units in the UK will have difficulty in implementing this degree of cover unless there is a substantial expansion in consultant numbers. In many countries where the lack of trained medical and midwifery staff is a reality, providing adequate intrapartum cover will undoubtedly be difficult. In such settings trained health or birth attendants may be an alternative. Regular training of these personnel to recognise intrapartum problems and perhaps transfer of the mother to a regional, better-equipped unit may help in reducing perinatal and maternal complications.

Service modelling and care pathways

Key features of service modelling in high-risk obstetrics include an assessment of the accessibility, safety, effectiveness and efficiency of the service within an integrated national or regional maternity provision framework and must be supported by adequate funding. The views of the service providers (obstetricians and midwives) as well as consumers (pregnant women) must be incorporated when the service is developed. Other important factors include a pathway for the development of policies and protocols (clinical and nonclinical), budget management, coordination and integration of data information systems, recruitment of medical and midwifery staff and clinical governance. Service modelling will also necessarily involve liaison with other service providers both within and outside the specialty. Clearly, clinical care pathways will evolve from the complexity of the case mix seen in any particular institution or region, but they must be based on available resources and should be based on good evidence.

Auditable standards

The relevant Royal Colleges have produced 30 standards for maternity care.[15] Standard 12 relates primarily to intrapartum care. Its key points include the need for a robust and transparent clinical governance framework, effective multidisciplinary teamwork and good communication as an indicator of good clinical practice. In addition, there should be close monitoring of staffing levels and regular review of clinical and organisational protocols. Continuing professional development for all staff must be available. There should also be regular audit of clinical outcome. To facilitate implementation, each standard sets out specific auditable indicators and the process of audit against these standards will, it is hoped, act as one measure of safety. Where high standards are not achieved, data from audit may provide evidence to support a business case for additional resources.

Future research

In addition to basic scientific research into various maternal and fetal conditions, other areas of high-risk pregnancies that require further research include better methods of fetal monitoring, which would unequivocally reduce the incidence of birth asphyxia and the associated long-term morbidity. Better evidence regarding the optimal mode of delivery (for example, for multiple pregnancy) is also required, although the numbers required to provide clear guidance would be difficult to achieve outside a very large multicentre trial. A good example of this is the Term Breech Trial, which changed obstetric practice in a very short period of time.[17] Research into whether the model of perinatal care chosen for a particular country or region for high-risk pregnancies actually translates into improved outcomes is also needed.

Conclusions

Guidelines provide a framework from which healthcare providers can design clinical care pathways and organisational structures to improve care of the high-risk woman in labour. This invariably should reduce both maternal and fetal morbidity and mortality regardless of the healthcare setting.

References

1. Draper ES, Kurinczuk JJ, Lamming CR, Clarke M, James D, Field D. A confidential enquiry into cases of neonatal encephalopathy. *Arch Dis Child Fetal Neonatal Ed* 2002;87:F176–80.
2. Holt J, Fagerli I, Holdo B, Vold IN. Audit of neonatal deaths of nonmalformed infants of 34 weeks' gestation: unavoidable catastrophic events or suboptimal care? *Acta Obstet Gynecol Scand* 2002;81:899–904.
3. Jonsson M, Norden SL, Hanson U. Analysis of malpractice claims with a focus on oxytocin use in labour. *Acta Obstet Gynecol Scand* 2007;86:315–19.
4. Becher JC, Stenson BJ, Lyon AJ. Is intrapartum asphyxia preventable? *BJOG* 2007;114:1442–4.

5. Berglund S, Grunewald C, Pettersson H, Cnattingius S. Severe asphyxia due to delivery related malpractice in Sweden 1990–2005. *BJOG* 2008;115:316–23.
6. McClure EM, Saleem S, Pasha O, Goldenberg RL. Stillbirth in developing countries: a review of causes, risk factors and prevention strategies. *J Matern Fetal Neonatal Med* 2009;22:183–90.
7. Confidential Enquiry into Maternal and Child Health. *Perinatal Mortality 2007: England, Wales and Northern Ireland.* London: CEMACH 2009 [http://www.cmace.org.uk/getattachment/1d2c0ebc-d2aa-4131-98ed-56bf8269e529/Perinatal-Mortality-2007.aspx].
8. Jonsson M, Norden-Lindeberg S, Ostlund I, Hanson U. Metabolic acidosis at birth and suboptimal care-illustration of the gap between knowledge and clinical practice. *BJOG* 2009;116:1453–60.
9. Amer-Wahlin I, Hellsten C, Noren H, Hagberg H, Herbst A, Kjellmer I, et al. Cardiotocography only versus cardiotocography plus ST analysis of fetal electrocardiogram for intrapartum fetla monitoring: a Swedish randomised controlled trial. *Lancet* 2001;358:534–8.
10. Westgate J, Harris M, Curnow JS, Greene KR. Randomised trial of cardiotocography alone or with ST waveform analysis for intrapartum monitoring. *Lancet* 1992;340:194–8.
11. National Institute for Health and Clinical Excellence. *Intrapartum Care: Management and Delivery of Care to Women in Labour.* Clinical Guideline 55. London: NICE; 2007 [http://guidance.nice.org.uk/CG55].
12. Lewis G, editor. Saving Mothers' Lives: Reviewing Maternal Deaths to Make Motherhood Safer 2003–2005. The Seventh Report of the Confidential Enquiries into Maternal Deaths in the United Kingdom. London: CEMACH; 2007 [http://www.cmace.org.uk/getdoc/319fb647-d2c6-4b47-b6a0-a853a2f4de1b/Maternal-1.aspx].
13. NHS National Patient Safety Agency. *Seven Steps to Patient Safety. Full Reference Guide.* August 2004 [http://www.nrls.npsa.nhs.uk/resources/collections/seven-steps-to-patient-safety/?entryid45=59787].
14. Royal College of Obstetricians and Gynaecologists, Royal College of Anaesthetists, Royal College of Midwives and Royal College of Paediatrics and Child Health. *Safer Childbirth: Minimum Standards for the Organisation and Delivery of Care in Labour.* London; RCOG Press; 2007 [http://www.rcog.org.uk/womens-health/clinical-guidance/safer-childbirth-minimum-standards-organisation-and-delivery-care-la].
15. Royal College of Anaesthetists, Royal College of Midwives, Royal College of Obstetricians and Gynaecologists, Royal College of Paediatrics and Child Health. *Standards for Maternity Care. Report of a Working Party.* London: RCOG Press; 2008 [http://www.rcog.org.uk/womens-health/clinical-guidance/standards-maternity-care].
16. Royal College of Obstetrician and Gynaecologists. *The Future Role of the Consultant: A Working Party Report.* London: RCOG Press; 2005 [http://www.rcog.org.uk/womens-health/clinical-guidance/future-role-consultant].
17. Hannah ME, Hannah WJ, Hewson SA, Hodnett ED, Saigal S, Willan AR. Planned caesarean section versus planned vaginal birth for breech presentation at term: a randomised multi-centre trial. Term Breech Trial Collaborative Group. *Lancet* 2000;356:1375–83.

CHAPTER 12

Obesity in pregnancy

Jo Modder

Key points

✓ Women with maternal obesity and their babies are at high risk of specific adverse outcomes and require specific services and interventions.
✓ A number of interventions need to be carried out by primary care services before referral to the maternity services.
✓ Maternity services should develop a clinical care pathway for maternal obesity that takes into account locally agreed strategies for management.
✓ Dietetic services and weight management interventions may not be universally available and consideration needs to be given to how best to develop such services locally.
✓ The local organisation has responsibility for ensuring that health professionals involved in maternity care have access to appropriate education and training related to maternal obesity.
✓ Workforce planning should take the local prevalence of maternal obesity into consideration.

■ Introduction

The prevalence of obesity in the general population has increased markedly over the past few decades, accompanied by a parallel increase in the prevalence of obesity in pregnancy. Obesity in pregnancy is defined as a body mass index (BMI) of $30kg/m^2$ or more at the antenatal booking visit. There are three different classes of obesity:

● BMI 30.0–34.9 (class 1)
● BMI 35.0–39.9 (class 2)
● BMI 40 and over (class 3 or morbid obesity).

Two observational studies in the UK reported an increase in maternal obesity prevalence rates from 9.4–9.9% in the early 1990s to 16–18% in 2002/04.[1,2]

Pregnant women who are obese are at increased risk of miscarriage,[3] gestational diabetes,[4] pre-eclampsia,[5] venous thromboembolism,[6,7] dys - functional labour,[8] caesarean section,[9] postpartum haemorrhage and wound infections,[4] and they are less likely to initiate or maintain breast-feeding.[10] Babies whose mothers are obese are at increased risk of stillbirth,[11] congenital anomalies,[12] prematurity, macrosomia and neo - natal death.[13] Maternal obesity can cause significant technical difficulties with respect to fetal surveillance, patient transfer, anaesthesia, labour and delivery, and experienced healthcare professionals need to be involved in the provision of their care.

▓ National guidance and clinical guidelines

The Centre for Maternal and Child Enquiries (CMACE) in the UK has developed national consensus standards of care for women with maternal obesity and these are available to clinicians and commissioners as CMACE/RCOG guidance.[14] An American College of Obstetricians and Gynecologists (ACOG) Committee Opinion Paper made a number of recommendations for obesity in pregnancy, including the recording of maternal height and weight at the first prenatal visit, encouraging an exercise programme during pregnancy, screening for gestational diabetes and obtaining an antenatal anaesthetic review.[15] The National Institute for Health and Clinical Excellence (NICE) is developing a guideline on weight management during pregnancy, which is anticipated to be published in 2010.

▓ Services and care required for women who are obese before and during pregnancy

NICE recommends that managers and health professionals in all primary care settings should ensure that preventing and managing obesity is a priority at both strategic and delivery levels and that dedicated resources should be allocated for action.[16] Women with obesity who wish to become pregnant fall within this recommendation in terms of precon-ception care and advice, consideration of weight loss programmes prior to conception and screening for comorbidities.

As a minimum, the provision of care for women with obesity who are planning pregnancy should include the following:

- regular monitoring of weight and BMI
- provision of information about the risks of maternal obesity
- advice regarding how best to achieve weight loss prior to conception
- screening for comorbidities
- commencement of higher-dose (5 mg daily) folic acid supplementation (prevention of neural tube defects).

Regular monitoring of weight and BMI will identify women at risk and enable appropriate advice and weight loss interventions. A large observational study has shown that weight gain between pregnancies is linearly associated with the risk of pre-eclampsia, gestational diabetes, large-for-gestational-age babies, caesarean section and stillbirth.[17]

For women who are obese and already pregnant, the minimum requirements for the provision of care include:

- appropriate facilities and equipment available in all settings where maternity care is provided
- an agreed referral pathway for antenatal care
- provision of information to women regarding the potential risks of obesity and pregnancy and strategies to minimise risks
- a plan for antenatal care
- timely referral for appropriate specialist input (such as diet and lifestyle advice, anaesthesia and obstetric review)
- appropriately trained health professionals.

NICE obesity guidance recommends that any specialist setting should be equipped to care for people with obesity, including special seating (such as extra-wide chairs without arms), beds and adequate weighing and monitoring equipment.[16] In the maternity care setting, this includes extra-wide delivery beds and operating theatre tables with appropriate safe working loads.

The antenatal care plan should, as a minimum, include risk assessment for thromboprophylaxis, referral for dietary advice by an appropriately trained health professional,[18] screening for gestational diabetes and pre-eclampsia, obstetric review to discuss management of labour and delivery and anaesthetic assessment to identify any potential difficulties of intravenous access and regional and general anaesthesia.

█ Service models and clinical care pathways

There is debate as to whether maternity services should establish specialist multidisciplinary antenatal clinics for maternal obesity or whether care of these women should be integrated into all antenatal clinics, with clear guidelines for care made available. The former option requires extra resource in terms of venue, clinical and administrative staffing, while the latter option requires all health professionals to be aware of the possible adverse outcomes and the strategies to minimise them. Figure 12.1 shows an example of a clinical care pathway for pregnant women with maternal obesity.

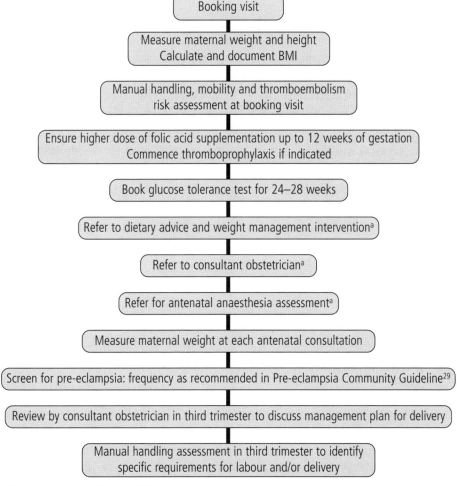

Figure 12.1 Example of a clinical care pathway for women with maternal obesity

[a] Depending on locally agreed pathway

Special issues related to service delivery

Measuring and recording maternal weight, height and BMI

The NICE antenatal care guideline recommends that maternal height and weight should be recorded for all women at the initial booking visit to allow the calculation of BMI.[19] There is evidence that self-reported rather than measured height and weight may be used at some booking visits, owing to lack of availability of appropriate equipment.[1] However, self-reported weight may be underestimated, leading to inaccurate risk assessment.[20]

Lifestyle and weight management interventions

An appropriately trained health professional should provide dietary counselling to women who are obese.[18] However, the CEMACH Diabetes Programme identified that 54% of women with type 1 and type 2 diabetes in England, Wales and Northern Ireland were seen by a dietician during pregnancy.[21] This suggests that there may be resource issues for dietetic services and local maternity services will need to decide how best to provide such advice to women during pregnancy.

There has recently been a revision to the 1990 Institute of Medicine guideline on weight gain in pregnancy and it is now recommended that women with a BMI of 30 or above should have a total pregnancy weight gain of 5–9 kg; if they are to achieve this target, women are likely to require weight management interventions during pregnancy.[22]

Women with obesity should have access to a referral pathway to appropriate healthcare professionals for supporting the adoption of a healthy lifestyle, including diet quality and physical activity patterns.[18]

Equipment and facilities

Current national guidance is that any specialist setting should have facilities to adequately care for people with obesity.[16] A UK-wide survey by the Centre for Maternal and Child Enquiries (CMACE) showed that maternity units did not consistently have such facilities (CMACE, unpublished data). Facilities and equipment include large blood-pressure cuffs, extra-large thromboembolic deterrent stockings and theatre gowns and extra-wide chairs, wheelchairs and transfer trolleys.

Training

The education of health professionals concerning the impact of maternal obesity on maternal and fetal outcomes should be incorporated into continuing education programmes for the different disciplines involved in providing care. The joint Royal Colleges *Safer Childbirth* standards document highlights the responsibility of the local organisation to ensure that all professional staff have the opportunity for in-service education and training sessions.[23] This could take the form of educational sessions on maternal obesity, including pregnancy outcomes and management.

Staffing and manpower planning

Senior obstetric input

Women with maternal obesity have a higher risk of comorbidities and require an agreed management plan for delivery made at senior level in partnership with the woman. A consultant obstetrician should be immediately available for caesarean section in a woman with a BMI greater than 40.[24]

Midwifery care during labour

Women with maternal obesity fall into category V of the case-mix classification used by the Birthrate Plus workforce planning tool, which needs a ratio of 1.4 whole-time equivalent midwives to one woman.[25] Maternity services will need to identify the prevalence of maternal obesity within the local maternity unit population to ensure adequate midwifery workforce planning.

Obstetric anaesthesia cover for the labour ward

Maternal obesity can present serious technical difficulties to the anaesthetist and women may present to the service in an emergency situation. Intravenous access and regional and general anaesthesia for these women may require an anaesthetist who is suitably experienced: the duty anaesthetist for the labour ward must have access to prompt assistance from a consultant anaesthetist whenever required.[18]

■ Audit

Maternity units should carry out regular audits of practice against locally agreed standards for women with obesity in pregnancy. The minimum requirements to achieve level 3 of standard 3: criterion 10 (obesity in pregnancy) within the NHSLA Clinical Negligence Scheme for Trusts (CNST) include the following:

● audit of the calculation and documentation of BMI for all women receiving maternity care
● monitoring whether an antenatal assessment with an obstetric anaesthetist has been offered
● monitoring whether the availability of suitable equipment in all care settings for women with a high BMI has been assessed at local level.[26]

Minimum key indicators to measure efficiency and safety of care are suggested below:

● percentage of women booking for antenatal care who have maternal weight, maternal height and BMI recorded
● percentage of women booking for antenatal care who have a BMI of 30 or above
● percentage of women with a booking BMI of 30 or above who commenced 5 mg folic acid supplementation prior to conception
● percentage of women with a booking BMI of 30 or above who have a documented risk assessment of venous thromboembolism at the booking visit[27]
● percentage of maternity staff who have had training in manual handling techniques and the use of specialist bariatric equipment within the previous 12 months
● percentage of women with a BMI equivalent to or greater than the locally agreed threshold who have had an anaesthesia assessment during the antenatal period
● percentage of women with a booking BMI of 30 or above who had a glucose tolerance test during pregnancy[28]
● percentage of operative vaginal deliveries and caesarean sections in women with morbid obesity (booking BMI of 40 or above) that were attended by an obstetrician and anaesthetist at specialty trainee level 6 or above.

Future research

Areas requiring further research have been identified by a number of organisations; the key topics are:

- the optimal weight gain during pregnancy for women in different BMI categories
- the optimal caesarean section technique for women with obesity in pregnancy
- the perceptions of women with obesity in pregnancy regarding their interactions with healthcare services
- the effects of diet and lifestyle interventions during pregnancy on maternal and fetal outcomes
- the optimal gestation for screening women with maternal obesity for impaired glucose tolerance
- the clinical benefit of low-dose aspirin during pregnancy for women with morbid obesity.

References

1. Heslehurst N, Ells LJ, Simpson H, Batterham A, Wilkinson J, Summerbell CD. Trends in maternal obesity incidence rates, demographic predictors, and health inequalities in 36,821 women over a 15-year period. *BJOG* 2007;114:187–94.
2. Kanagalingam MG, Forouhi NG, Greer IA, Sattar N. Changes in booking body mass index over a decade: retrospective analysis from a Glasgow Maternity Hospital. *BJOG* 2005;112:1431–3.
3. Lashen H, Fear K, Sturdee DW. Obesity is associated with increased risk of first trimester and recurrent miscarriage: matched case–control study. *Hum Reprod* 2002;19:1644–6.
4. Sebire NJ, Jolly M, Harris JP, Wadsworth J, Joffe M, Beard RW, et al. Maternal obesity and pregnancy outcome: a study of 287,213 pregnancies in London. *Int J Obes Relat Metab Disord* 2001;25:1175–82.
5. O'Brien TE, Ray JG, Chan WS. Maternal body mass index and the risk of preeclampsia: a systematic overview. *Epidemiology* 2003;14:368–74.
6. Larsen TB, Sørensen HT, Gislum M, Johnsen SP. Maternal smoking, obesity, and risk of venous thromboembolism during pregnancy and the puerperium: a population-based nested case–control study. *Thromb Res* 2007;120:505–9.
7. Jacobsen AF, Skjeldestad FE, Sandset PM. Ante- and postnatal risk factors of venous thrombosis: a hospital-based case control study. *J Thromb Haemost* 2008;6:905–12.
8. Nuthalapaty FS, Rouse DJ, Owen J. The association of maternal weight with cesarean risk, labor duration, and cervical dilation rate during labor induction. *Obstet Gynecol* 2004;103:452–6. Erratum in *Obstet Gynecol* 2004;103:1019.
9. Chu SY, Kim SY, Schmid CH, Dietz PM, Callaghan WM, Lau J, et al. Maternal obesity and risk of cesarean delivery: a meta-analysis. *Obes Rev* 2007;8:385–94.

10. Amir LH, Donath S. A systematic review of maternal obesity and breastfeeding intention, initiation and duration. *BMC Pregnancy Childbirth* 2007;7:9.

11. Chu SY, Kim SY, Lau J, Schmid CH, Dietz PM, Callaghan WM, et al. Maternal obesity and risk of stillbirth: a meta-analysis. *Am J Obstet Gynecol* 2007;197:223–8.

12. Rasmussen SA, Chu SY, Kim SY, Schmid CH, Lau J. Maternal obesity and risk of neural tube defects: a meta-analysis. *Am J Obstet Gynecol* 2008;198:611–9.

13. Cedergren MI. Maternal morbid obesity and the risk of adverse pregnancy outcome. *Obstet Gynecol* 2008;103:219–24.

14. Centre for Maternal and Child Enquiries; Royal College of Obstetricians and Gynaecologists. *Management of Women with Obesity in Pregnancy*. CMACE/RCOG Joint Guideline. London: CMACE; 2010 [http://www.rcog.org.uk/womens-health/clinical-guidance/management-women-obesity-pregnancy].

15. American College of Obstetricians and Gynecologists, Committee on Gynecologic Practice. ACOG Committee Opinion number 315. Obesity and pregnancy. *Obstet Gynecol* 2005;106:671–5.

16. National Institute for Health and Clinical Excellence. *Obesity: Guidance on the Prevention, Identification, Assessment and Management of Overweight and Obesity in Adults and Children*. London: NICE; 2006 [http://www.nice.org.uk/nicemedia/pdf/CG43NICEGuideline.pdf]

17. Villamor E, Cnattingius S. Interpregnancy weight change and risk of adverse pregnancy outcomes: a population-based study. *Lancet* 2006;368:1164–70.

18. Royal College of Obstetrics and Gynaecology. Consensus views arising from the 53rd Study Group: Obesity and Reproductive Health. In: Baker P, Balen A, Poston L, Sattar N, editors. *Obesity and Reproductive Health*. London: RCOG Press; 2007. p. 271–4 [http://www.rcog.org.uk/womens-health/clinical-guidance/obesity-and-reproductive-health-study-group-statement].

19. National Institute for Health and Clinical Excellence. *Antenatal Care: Routine Care for the Healthy Pregnant Woman*. NICE Clinical Guideline 62. London: NICE; 2008 [http://guidance.nice.org.uk/CG62].

20. Gorber SC, Tremblay M, Moher D, Gorber B. A comparison of direct vs. self-report measures for assessing height, weight and body mass index: a systematic review. *Obes Rev* 2007;8:373–4.

21. Confidential Enquiry into Maternal and Child Health. Diabetes in Pregnancy: Are We Providing the Best Care? Findings of a National Enquiry: February 2007 England, Wales and Northern Ireland. London: CEMACH; 2007 [http://www.cmace.org.uk/getattachment/ce7b601d-9a14-443e-982c-bcda4fd92ca3/Diabetes-in-Pregnancy.aspx].

22. Institute of Medicine. *Weight Gain During Pregnancy: Re-examining the Guidelines*. Washington DC: National Academies Press; 2009.

23. Royal College of Obstetricians and Gynaecologists, Royal College of Anaesthetists, Royal College of Midwives and Royal College of Paediatrics and Child Health. *Safer Childbirth: Minimum Standards for the Organisation and Delivery of Care in Labour*. London; RCOG Press; 2007 [http://www.rcog.org.uk/womens-health/clinical-guidance/safer-childbirth-minimum-standards-organisation-and-delivery-care-la].

24. Royal College of Obstetricians and Gynaecologists. *Responsibility of Consultant On Call*. Good Practice No. 8. London: RCOG; 2009 [http://www.rcog.org.uk/responsibility-of-consultant-on-call].

25. Ball JA, Washbrook M. *Birthrate Plus: A Framework for Workforce Planning and Decision-making for Maternity Services*. Hale, Cheshire: Books for Midwives; 1996.
26. NHS Litigation Authority. Clinical Negligence Scheme for Trusts: Maternity Clinical Risk Management Standards Version 1 2010/11 [http://www.nhsla.com/News/#{A0A8EE5C-A421-4925-AD44-6DF4E3ED8DDC}].
27. Royal College of Obstetricians and Gynaecologists. *Reducing the Risk of Thrombosis and Embolism During Pregnancy and the Puerperium*. Green-Top Guideline No. 37. London: RCOG; 2009 [http://www.rcog.org.uk/womens-health/clinical-guidance/reducing-risk-of-thrombosis-greentop37].
28. National Institute for Health and Clinical Excellence. *Diabetes in Pregnancy: Management of Diabetes and its Complications From Pre-Conception to the Postnatal Period*. London: NICE; 2008 [http://guidance.nice.org.uk/CG63].
29. Action on Pre-eclampsia. *PRECOG: The Pre-eclampsia Community Guideline*. London: APEC; 2004 [http://www.apec.org.uk/precog.htm].

CHAPTER 13

Prevention of hypoxic ischaemic encephalopathy

Osric Navti and Justin Konje

Key points

✓ Current approaches for the prevention of hypoxic ischaemic encephalopathy include antenatal identification and monitoring of fetal growth restriction and electronic fetal monitoring accompanied by intrapartum fetal blood sampling.

✓ Intrapartum monitoring of the fetal heart rate remains the most commonly used tool for identification of an at-risk fetus and allows for timely intervention.

✓ All units should have a regular continuing programme of in-service training, including cardiotocograph interpretation, drills on emergency caesarean section and neonatal resuscitation.

■ Introduction

Hypoxic ischaemic encephalopathy (HIE) is defined as neonatal enceph - alopathy associated with intrapartum hypoxia in the absence of any other abnormality.[1] Neonatal encephalopathy is defined clinically as disturbed neurological function in the infant at or near term during the first week after birth, manifested by difficulties with initiating and maintaining respiration, depression of tone and reflexes, altered level of consciousness and, often, seizures.[2]

It has been suggested that 2–8/1000 term infants suffer from neonatal encephalopathy of any aetiology. The precise incidence of HIE is, how - ever, unknown, largely because previously it was assumed that all cases of HIE resulted from intrapartum asphyxia. There has been increasing evidence that only a small proportion of cases of HIE are secondary to intrapartum events. These vary from 10% of all HIE to 1.6/10 000 births.[3] Data from a prospective national collaborative perinatal project study in the USA demonstrated that approximately 9% of cases of cerebral palsy were attributable to possible birth asphyxia.[4] As tech - nology advances, it should be easier to distinguish between HIE primarily from intrapartum asphyxia and that secondary to other factors, some of which may be aggravated by intrapartum events. In a retrospective case–control study in Perth, Australia, it was observed that approxi- mately 33% of babies with HIE had only antenatal risk factors, 25% had both antepartum and evidence of intrapartum hypoxia, 4% had evidence of intrapartum hypoxia in the absence of preconceptual or antepartum factors and 2% had no recognised risk factors. The strongest antepartum risk factor was fetal growth restriction (FGR).

In 1999, the International Cerebral Palsy Task Force published its consensus statement specifying the criteria for the definition of an acute intrapartum event sufficient to cause HIE. These criteria were endorsed by the American College of Obstetricians and Gynecologists Task Force on Neonatal Encephalopathy and Cerebral Palsy in 2003.[1] These groups agree that, to diagnose HIE as secondary to acute intrapartum events, the following essential criteria have to be fulfilled:

- evidence of a metabolic acidosis in fetal umbilical artery cord blood obtained at delivery (pH less than 7.00 and base deficit 12 mmol/l or greater)
- early onset of severe or moderate neonatal encephalopathy in infants 34 weeks or more of gestation
- cerebral palsy of the spastic quadriplegia or dyskinetic type
- exclusion of other identifiable aetiology such as trauma, coagulation disorders, infectious conditions or genetic disorders.

Criteria that collectively suggest an intrapartum timing (within close proximity to labour and delivery; for example, 0–48 hours) but are non - specific to asphyxia are:

- a sentinel (signal) hypoxic event occurring immediately before or during labour
- a sudden and sustained fetal bradycardia or the absence of fetal heart variability in the presence of persistent late or variable decelerations, usually after a hypoxic sentinel event when the pattern was previously normal

- Apgar scores of 0–3 beyond 5 minutes
- onset of multisystem involvement within 72 hours of birth
- early imaging study showing evidence of acute nonfocal cerebral abnormality.

The birth of an infant who has a possible HIE is a source of great concern to the parents, obstetricians and paediatricians. Hypoxic cerebral brain injury that occurs in the perinatal period is recognised as a cause of severe long-term neurological deficit in children; it is often referred to as cerebral palsy.[4,5] Although care of the affected infant is the primary responsibility of the parent, it is of concern to all involved, as not only is the occurrence of HIE an adverse outcome but it also opens the door for possible litigation. In the UK, 20% of all claims are from obstetrics but 60% of payments relate to claims arising out of birth.[6] HIE is considered the single major contributor. This has resulted in scrutiny of intrapartum care by the Department of Health in the UK with the aim of reducing obstetric litigation by 25% in 2005.[7] Prevention of HIE is therefore not only an essential part of maternity care but one of the key standards by which units are judged for delivery of high-quality obstetrics care.

The prognosis for infants affected by HIE is determined by the stage of encephalopathy (Table 13.1) and the availability of neonatal expertise.

Table 13.1 Stages of neonatal encephalopathy[17] with subsequent long-term prognosis[18–20]

Stage of encephalopathy	Clinical signs	Likelihood of subsequent associated disability or infant death (%)
1: Mild	Hyperalertness Uninhibited primitive reflexes Sympathetic effects	Almost zero
2: Moderate	Obtundation Mild hypotonia Distal flexion Seizures	20–27
3: Severe	Stupor or coma Flaccidity Suppressed brain stem and autonomic function	50–72

What women want (surveys and commissioning advice)

Unfortunately, unlike most other areas of perinatal care, there are no local, national or international surveys on what women want with regard to HIE. However, it is reasonable to extrapolate that most women will require:

- a guarantee that healthcare providers will take all measures considered reasonable to minimise the risk of HIE
- that care providers will be familiar with those at risk of HIE and, consequently, will take appropriate steps to prevent intrapartum asphyxia, which may result in HIE
- that early warning signs of intrapartum asphyxia will be recognised and timely interventions instituted
- that neonatal facilities will be adequate and readily available to care for babies that have suffered from intrapartum asphyxia
- that appropriate levels of expertise will be available to recognise and deal with any immediate complications of birth, including possible HIE.

The absence of information and specific guidelines on HIE means that advice provided to women has to be collated from evidence-based effective antenatal and perinatal care that maximises the opportunity to deliver a healthy baby.

National and clinical guidance

Any guidelines will focus essentially on prevention and management of HIE. This cannot, however, be discussed without first identifying those at risk of HIE. Box 13.1 summarises these conditions. Not all risk factors carry the same magnitude of risk.

Prevention

Although several approaches have been suggested for the prevention of HIE, none is reliable and guarantees prevention. Current approaches include antenatal identification and monitoring of FGR and electronic fetal monitoring accompanied by intrapartum fetal blood sampling.

Antenatally the most important risk factor that should be identified is FGR. FGR is the failure of a fetus to achieve its growth potential; the majority but not all cases of FGR are also small for gestational age (SGA).

Box 13.1 Risk factors for hypoxic ischaemic encephalopathy

Maternal conditions
- Inflammatory conditions
  - Infection: maternal or placental (e.g. chorioamnionitis)
  - coagulopathy
- Maternal age – older mother
- Family history
- Hypertension
- Thyroid dysfunction
- Epilepsy
- Infertility
- Vaginal bleeding
- Poor socio-economic status

Intrapartum considerations
- Preterm birth
- Intrauterine infection
- Antepartum bleeding
- Acute sentinel events:
  - Ruptured uterus
  - Cord prolapsed
  - Placental abruption
  - Fetal exsanguination (vasa praevia)
  - Maternal cardiac arrest

Fetal factors
- Multiple pregnancies (highest risk in monochorionic twins)
- Preterm prelabour rupture of membranes
- Prelabour rupture of membranes
- Meconium-stained liquor
- Fetal growth restriction, especially when associated with intrauterine infection
- Macrosomia/large for gestational age at birth (≥ 4.5 kg at birth)
- Preterm birth
- Congenital or genetic anomalies

Although regular symphysiofundal height measurements are not highly sensitive in terms of identifying FGR, a combination of risk factor screening, uterine artery Doppler measurements and serial ultrasound fetal biometry could significantly reduce the number of cases of FGR unrecognised before delivery. Where the fetus at risk has been identified, planning for intrapartum care must be such that further insult from intrapartum asphyxia is minimised.

During labour, there is a relative oxygen deficiency and therefore a significant threat to the intact survival of the fetus. A healthy fetus should have the physiological ability to sustain even stressful labour without handicap, but this is often not the case if the fetus is already compromised or when a healthy fetus is subjected to exceptional hypoxic stress during labour. Intrapartum fetal monitoring is aimed at minimising such risks. The purpose of intrapartum monitoring is to ensure the delivery of a healthy baby by the most appropriate means without jeopardising the health of the mother. The challenge of monitoring is to identify fetuses whose defence mechanisms are compromised before permanent damage is sustained and to distinguish the effect of acute lack of oxygen in a healthy fetus from the same insult in an already compromised fetus.

Monitoring of the fetal heart rate intrapartum remains the most commonly used tool for identification of at-risk fetuses to allow for timely intervention. Such monitoring can be achieved by electronic fetal monitoring with computerised or noncomputerised cardiotocography (CTG), pulse oximetry, fetal auscultation (intermittent) with a stethoscope or Doppler device and STAN, which combines standard CTG technology with the unique fetal electrocardiogram ST analysis. Abnormal fetal heart rate patterns have a high false-positive rate and are a poor predictor of HIE. For a previously normal fetus, HIE is most likely to follow a sentinel event such as cord prolapse, ruptured uterus, placental abruption, fetal exsanguination as occurs in cases of significant fetomaternal haemorrhage or rupture, vasa praevia and shoulder dystocia. The National Institute for Health and Clinical Excellence guideline on intrapartum care provides the definition and criteria for the identification of abnormalities with electronic fetal monitoring and suggested action.[8] This guidance is summarised in Tables 13.2 and 13.3.

Other approaches to the prevention of HIE include the antenatal administration of corticosteroids to women in preterm labour, as this has been shown to reduce perinatal mortality, respiratory distress and intraventricular haemorrhage by over 50%.[8] Potential intrapartum

Table 13.2 Definition of normal, suspicious and pathological fetal heart rate traces

Category	Definition
Normal	A trace in which all four features are classified as reassuring
Suspicious	A trace with one feature classified as nonreassuring and the remaining features classified as reassuring
Pathological	A trace with two or more features classified as nonreassuring or one or more classified as abnormal

Table 13.3 Classification of fetal heart rate trace features

Feature	Baseline (beats/ minute)	Variability (bpm)	Decelerations	Accelerations
Reassuring	110–160	≥5	None	Present
Nonreassuring	100–109 161–180	<5 for 40–90 mins	Typical variable decelerations with over 50% of contractions, occurring for over 90 minutes Single prolonged deceleration for up to 3 minutes	The absence of accelerations with otherwise normal trace is of uncertain significance
Abnormal	<100 >180 Sinusoidal pattern ≥10 mins	<5 for 90 mins	Either atypical variable decelerations with over 50% of contractions or late decelerations, both for over 30 minutes Single prolonged deceleration for more than 3 minutes	

measures include the use of beta 2 agonists such as terbutaline in cases of uterine hyperstimulation and intrapartum hypoxia and the appropriate use of fetal blood sampling to identify fetal acidosis and then urgently expediting delivery.

The NICE guideline on intrapartum care lists factors whose presence should suggest a planned birth in an obstetric unit.[8] These include multiple birth, placenta praevia, pre-eclampsia or pregnancy-induced hypertension, preterm labour or preterm prelabour rupture of membranes, placental abruption, recurrent antepartum haemorrhage, small for gestational age in this pregnancy (less than fifth centile or reduced growth velocity on ultrasound), abnormal fetal heart rate (FHR)/Doppler studies and ultrasound diagnosis of oligohydramnios or polyhydramnios.

The guidelines also recommend changing from intermittent auscultation to continuous electronic fetal monitoring in low-risk women where there is:

- significant meconium-stained liquor (this change should also be considered for light meconium-stained liquor)
- abnormal FHR detected by intermittent auscultation (less than 110 beats/minute; greater than 160 beats/minute; any decelerations after a contraction)
- maternal pyrexia (defined as 38.0°C once or 37.5°C on two occasions 2 hours apart)
- fresh vaginal bleeding in labour
- oxytocin use for augmentation
- a request by the woman.

Most of the factors highlighted above are associated with an increased risk of HIE and therefore call for increased surveillance.

Special issues related to service delivery

Labour ward staffing

Research has demonstrated a high prevalence of suboptimal intrapartum care among cases of perinatal death in the UK: in one series, the suboptimal care involved professionals in 96% of encephalopathy cases.[9] This has prompted a reassessment of labour ward management with the aim of improving pregnancy outcomes.[10] There is also some evidence suggesting that training in obstetric emergencies within a UK unit resulted in a significant reduction in low 5-minute Apgar scores and HIE. The improvement was sustained as the training continued.[11] Observational data from a large Scottish perinatal centre demonstrated a marked reduction in the incidence of asphyxia-related mortality and morbidity over a 12-year period. Possible explanations offered for this were the transfer of delivery unit leadership to a small group of specialist high-risk obstetricians and developments in clinical practice such as universal training in CTG implementation and a programme of clinical risk management. It was, however, noted that the decline in asphyxia-related mortality and morbidity preceded these service developments.[12]

A Healthcare Commission review of maternity services in the UK highlighted several concerns in some trusts. These included staffing levels falling well below recommended levels, inadequate consultant presence on labour wards, poor in-house training for doctors and midwives, poor adherence to recommended guidelines and poor communication.[13] In *Safer Childbirth*, minimum standards for the organisation and delivery of care in labour are set out.[14] This report recommends increasing consultant presence on labour wards to over 100 hours a week in units delivering over 5000 babies annually.[14]

Neonatal networks and neonatal intensive care services

The reorganisation of care into neonatal networks has improved the coordination and consistency of services, pointing to increased effectiveness. There are, however, still serious capacity and staffing problems and a lack of clear data on outcomes. Neonatal services are part of a continuum of care that starts with maternity services, but they are at present commissioned and planned separately rather than as part of a whole systems approach. There is a need for targeted research aimed at reducing the demand for neonatal care through improved understanding and prevention of the trigger factors associated with preterm birth, low birth weight and sickness in newborns. The British Association for Perinatal Medicine provides standards for hospitals supplying neonatal intensive and high-dependency care.[15] It makes clear that all maternity hospitals, including those that do not provide intensive or high-dependency care, must have staff and facilities for resuscitation and stabilisation for the unexpectedly sick newborn infant; hospitals providing neonatal intensive and high-dependency care must have continuous availability of qualified medical and nursing staff and resources to meet the needs of all babies. There must be agreed procedures for the transfer of high-risk obstetric cases and the postnatal transfer of sick babies.

Criteria for a paediatric presence in the delivery suite should include cases with significant fetal distress, preterm deliveries, likelihood of severe fetal compromise, babies with major fetal anomalies and all 'crash call' deliveries.

Training

There is clear evidence of improvement in neonatal outcomes with obstetric emergency training.[11] Developments in clinical practice, such as universal training in CTG interpretation and a programme of clinical risk management, have been suggested as reasons for a reduction in the number of cases of intrapartum asphyxia.[12] All units should therefore have a regular continuing programme of in-service training including CTG interpretation, drills on emergency ('crash') caesarean section and neonatal resuscitation.[16] In addition, the staff of each unit should attend regular multidisciplinary meetings with midwives, obstetricians and pathologists to be aware of trends in mortality and morbidity. Nurses, midwives and doctors must be able to demonstrate continuing professional development.

Future research

Research is needed into the impact of new electronic fetal monitoring interventions on the occurrence of HIE.

Audit

Auditable standards include:

- decision to delivery interval for 'crash' emergency caesarean section
- umbilical cord blood gas analysis for all emergency deliveries
- confidential reviews of the management of all cases of HIE
- all infants with moderate or severe encephalopathy should have a psychometric assessment at 18 months of age.

References

1. American College of Obstetricians and Gynecologists Task Force on Neonatal Encephalopathy and Cerebral Palsy; American Academy of Pediatrics. *Neonatal Encephalopathy and Cerebal Palsy: Defining the Pathogenesis and Pathophysiology.* Washington, DC: ACOG; 2003.
2. MacLennan A. A template for defining a causal relation between acute intrapartum events and cerebral palsy: international consensus statement. *BMJ* 1999;319:1054–9.
3. Badawi N, Kurinczuk JJ, Keogh JM, Alessandri LM, O'Sullivan F, Burton PR, et al. Intrapartum risk factors for newborn encephalopathy: the Western Australian case–control study. *BMJ* 1998;317:1554–8.

4. Perlman JM. Intrapartum hypoxic ischemic injury and subsequent cerebral palsy: medicolegal issues. *Pediatrics* 1997;99:851–9.
5. Volpe JJ. Hypoxic-ischemic encephalopathy. In: Volpe JJ, editor. *Neurology of the Newborn*. Philadelphia, PA: WB Saunders; 2001. p. 277–95.
6. NHS Litigation Authority. Claims. Factsheet 5 2008/09 [http://www.nhsla.com/claims].
7. Department of Health. An Organisation With a Memory: Report of an Expert Group on Learning From Adverse Events in the NHS. London: TSO; 2000.
8. National Institute for Health and Clinical Excellence. *Intrapartum Care: Management and Delivery of Care to Women in Labour*. Clinical Guideline 55. London: NICE; 2007 [http://guidance.nice.org.uk/CG55].
9. Draper ES, Kurinezuk JJ, Lamming CR, James D, Field D. A confidential enquiry into cases of neonatal encephalopathy. *Arch Dis Child Fetal Neonatal Ed* 2002;87:F176–80.
10. Papworth S, Cartlidge P. Learning from adverse events: the role of confidential enquiries. *Semin Fetal Neonatal Med* 2005;10:39–43.
11. Draycott T, Sibanda T, Owen L, Akande V, Winter C, Reading S, et al. Does training in obstetric emergencies improve neonatal outcome? *BJOG* 2006;113:177–82.
12. Becher J, Stenson B, Lyon A. Is intrapartum asphyxia preventable? *BJOG* 2007;114:1442–4.
13. Healthcare Commission. *Towards Better Births. A Review of Maternity Services in England*. London: Commission for Healthcare Audit and Inspection; 2008 [http://www.cqc.org.uk/publications.cfm?fde_id=625].
14. Royal College of Obstetricians and Gynaecologists, Royal College of Anaesthetists, Royal College of Midwives and Royal College of Paediatrics and Child Health. *Safer Childbirth: Minimum Standards for the Organisation and Delivery of Care in Labour*. London; RCOG Press; 2007 [http://www.rcog.org.uk/womens-health/clinical-guidance/safer-childbirth-minimum-standards-organisation-and-delivery-care-la].
15. British Association of Perinatal Medicine. Standards for Hospitals Providing Neonatal Intensive and High Dependency Care. (Second Edition) and Categories of Babies requiring Neonatal Care. 2001. London: BAPM; 2001 [http://www.bapm.org/publications].
16. British Paediatric Association. *Neonatal Resuscitation: Report of a BPA Working Party*. London; BPA; 1993.
17. Samat HB, Samat MS. Neonatal encephalopathy following fetal distress: a clinical and electroencephalographic study. *Arch Neurol* 1976;33:696–705.
18. Low JA. Intrapartum fetal asphyxia: definition, diagnosis and classification. *Am J Obstet Gynecol* 1997;176:957–9.
19. Low JA. Galbraith RS, Muir DW, Killen HL, Pater EA, Karchmar EJ. The relationship between perinatal hypoxia and newborn encephalopathy. *Am J Obstet Gynecol* 1985;152:256–60.
20. Dixon G, Badawi N, Kurinczuk JJ, Keogh JM, Silburn SR, Zubrick SR, et al. Early developmental outcomes after newborn encephalopathy. *Pediatrics* 2002;109:26–33.

CHAPTER 14

Risk management on the labour ward

Sonia Barnfield and Tim Draycott

Key points

- ✓ Labour can be a risky business.
- ✓ Risk management should be system-based.
- ✓ Risk management improves patient safety, which is important to women.
- ✓ There are emerging examples of risk management-led interventions to improve safety, such as the RCOG Maternity Dashboard.
- ✓ Training and system improvements may be the most effective interventions after adverse events.
- ✓ Research should aim to develop effective, generalisable risk management tools that could be made easily available to all units.

▊ Introduction

Labour and delivery can be a risky business; up to 8% of deliveries are complicated by a suboptimal outcome.[1] Enquiries into suboptimal outcomes have identified common and recurring errors including:

- failure to recognise problems
- confusion in roles and responsibilities
- failure to prioritise and perform clinical tasks in a structured, coordinated manner
- poor communication
- lack of organisational support.[2,3]

Risk management was initially developed to reduce the high litigation costs in medicine. Obstetric claims currently represent 20% of all claims dealt with by the UK National Health Service Litigation Authority (NHSLA), but 60% of payments relate to claims arising out of birth.[4] Legal claims in cases of cerebral palsy arising from negligent intrapartum care account for most of the NHS's annual litigation bill. However the focus of risk management has changed to improve the quality of patient care, which should consequentially avoid and reduce claims.[5]

Risk management aims to reduce poor outcomes by first identifying adverse events, creating a database to identify common patterns and developing a system of accountability to prevent future incidents.[5]

Reactive risk management has been highlighted in the case of Northwick Park Hospital, North West London, where ten maternal deaths occurred in a 3-year period. Two Healthcare Commission reports found that, as well as active failures, there were many latent conditions that played a role in many of the deaths: lack of clinical leadership, poor relations between staff, inadequate cover of consultants, shortage of midwives and a lack of high-risk services.[6] Since this report, Northwick Park Hospital has improved outcomes after employing the Royal College of Obstetricians and Gynaecologists' (RCOG) risk management process.

There has been at least one other report of the RCOG risk management paradigm directly improving outcome[7] and there are many other indirect examples; risk management is an essential component of a modern labour ward.

What women want

A number of national organisations are concerned with safety in maternity care, including the Care Quality Commission, the Centre for Maternal and Child Enquiries (CMACE), NHSLA, the National Patient Safety Agency (NPSA) and the RCOG. Despite the plethora of standards and advice produced, the only government target for maternity is linked to choice rather than safety.[8] By contrast, women appear to value safety over choice. In a study to explore women's decision making surrounding vaginal or caesarean delivery, it was found that, while many women support the principle of choice, all women thought that concerns about their baby's or their own health should take precedence over personal preference.[9]

Safety has also been highlighted in other national reports and recommendations. The King's Fund set up an independent panel in 2007 to review the safety of NHS maternity services in England.[10] The panel concluded that:

- the overwhelming majority of births in England are safe; however, some births are less safe than they could be
- safety is the responsibility of each and every member of all the teams working in and supporting maternity services: not only midwives and obstetricians but also anaesthetists, support staff, managers and trust boards
- 'safe teams' are the key to improving the safety of maternity services.[10]

The *Safer Childbirth* report focuses on improving the safety and quality of maternity by following ten key areas of care provision, which includes having a robust and transparent clinical governance framework.[11] The National Childbirth Trust welcomed this report and considered that, if it were implemented, the report would bring improvements to the safety of maternity care and quality of care and great benefits to women, their children and their families.[12]

National guidance and clinical guidelines

One facet of risk management is the measurement of adverse events and this has been recognised by Lord Darzi. He recognised that safety cannot be improved if it cannot be measured. There are national standards for safety in maternity care that have been produced jointly by the Royal Colleges (see chapter 1).[13] To monitor these standards and any adverse events, the report recommended the use of the RCOG Maternity Dashboard.[14] The Maternity Dashboard is a tool that can be used to benchmark activity and monitor performance against locally agreed standards on a monthly basis so that appropriate actions can be taken. It can also provide information about latent conditions, such as staffing levels and numbers of confinements booked. Four categories are suggested: clinical activity, workforce, clinical outcomes and risk incidents or complaints. Each maternity unit, however, can adapt it to suit their needs. Individual units set goals for the parameters as well as upper and lower thresholds. A traffic light system is used: green when the goals are met, amber when they are above the lower threshold but not above the upper threshold indicating actions need to be taken, and red when the upper threshold is breached, requiring immediate action.

There have been calls for robust systems for monitoring healthcare outcomes and with the increasing use of electronic patient records in health care, there is an opportunity for the development and application of real-time monitoring systems that can lead to the rapid detection of adverse trends in healthcare, which in turn should lead to timely corrective action using standard risk management principles.[15] Best practice should improve care and clinical guidelines have been developed to promote best practice, reduce variation in care and improve outcomes.

The National Institute for Health and Clinical Excellence (NICE) has published many guidelines to promote best care (www.nice.org.uk). Other examples of national guidelines are those produced by the RCOG and the Scottish Intercollegiate Guidelines Network (www.sign. ac.uk). Although there are many national guidelines available, it is important that local units adapt these guidelines specifically for use in their unit, using the resources, staffing, medications and equipment available to them.

■ Service modelling and care pathways

Care bundles have been developed to make guidelines work 'at the coalface'. They can be complex or simple. An example of proactive risk management is the design of a cardiotocography (CTG) interpretation sticker,[16] a simple example that aids implementation of the NICE guideline. Since the implementation of a CTG sticker with targeted training, one unit has shown a 51% reduction in 5-minute Apgar scores less than 7 and a 50% reduction in HIE.[16] This is an example of a system approach where the system is improved to make the right way the easiest way. Humans are fallible; as Reason said, 'We cannot change the human condition but we can change the conditions under which humans work', so proactive risk management can improve safety by improving systems.[17]

Defences, barriers and safeguards occupy a key position in the system approach and form the 'Swiss cheese' model.[17] However, like Swiss cheese, these barriers can contain holes at certain times. These holes may arise for two reasons: active failures (unsafe acts committed by people, such as slips, lapses or procedural violations)[18] and latent conditions (such as staffing levels, inadequate equipment and staff skill mix). Latent conditions may lie dormant within the system for many years before they combine with active failures to create an accident opportunity. These latent conditions can be identified and remedied before an adverse event occurs, which can lead us towards proactive rather than reactive risk management.[17]

Reactive risk management can be examplified by the following flow diagram of one unit's experiences with CTG interpretation (Figure 14.1).

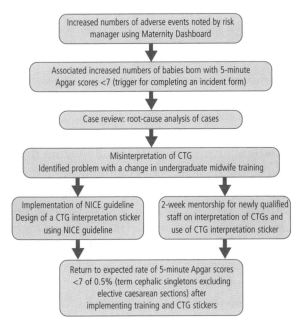

Figure 14.1 One unit's experiences with cardiotocography (CTG) interpretations

■ Special issues related to service delivery

Staffing of the labour ward may be the single most important risk. The Healthcare Commission's report *Towards Better Births*, a review of maternity services in England, found that staffing issues remain a significant factor in the delivery of safe maternity services.[19] With the introduction of the Working Time Regulations in August 2009 it is even more essential to increase consultant staffing to ensure the best training opportunities and supervision for junior doctors, as appropriate numbers of staff underpin a safe and quality service.[19]

Safer Childbirth recommends that 'women in established labour should receive individual one-to-one care from a midwife'.[11] This recommendation will help to promote and achieve greater levels of normality and the recommendation has also been endorsed by the National Childbirth Trust.[12]

Birthrate Plus (www.birthrateplus.co.uk) is a tool for assessing midwifery staffing that can identify shortfalls. Healthcare trusts collect a large sample of data on births related to their complexity, ranging from a simple, straightforward birth to emergency caesarean section, and the average birth time is measured. As births become more complex, more staff will be required.

Training

Training may be the single most effective part of system implementation for reactive and proactive risk management. The King's Fund reiterated this finding in their recommendation: 'Simulation-based training which assesses clinical, communication and team skills within a single exercise should be offered to all maternity staff, ideally within their own units'.[10]

CMACE has also highlighted poor communication and team working within multiprofessional obstetric and midwifery teams. The RCOG, RCM and CMACE have all recommended regular drill training in obstetric emergency management in the UK. This is now mandated by the Maternity Clinical Negligence Scheme for Trusts (CNST).[4] In particular, they advise training for cord prolapse, vaginal breech delivery, shoulder dystocia, eclampsia and antepartum and postpartum haemorrhage.

Training for staff in the core skills needed to handle emergency situations makes an important contribution to safety, although *Towards Better Births* found that there was a wide variation in trusts' training programmes, including the multiprofessional nature and attendance levels.[19] Currently, there is no national standard for the provision of training in the UK and, although regular training is recommended, few training programmes have been described in the literature and even fewer training programmes have been evaluated.[20]

'Teams that work together should also train together, with regular training taking place on the labour ward rather than on "away days" and being seen as a core activity rather than an optional extra.'[10] However, not all training is equal. In two cities in the South of England, training for shoulder dystocia started as a response to CNST in 2000, with very different results. In one city, a 70% reduction in brachial plexus injuries was demonstrated, while in another, a 100% increase in such injuries was demonstrated.[21,22]

Thus, not all training is 'good and effective training'. However, there are now several units that have demonstrated improved outcomes

(Kirkpatrick level 4)[23] and one review has identified common features in effective training programmes: institution-level incentives to train; a high participation rate with regular, multiprofessional in-house training; teamwork training integrated with clinical training; and the use of high-fidelity simulation models.[24]

Staffing and manpower planning

It is important to have a risk manager who has proper training and pro-tected time and, ideally, an enthusiastic and nonjudgemental approach. There should also be a dedicated labour ward consultant for risk management.[11] All staff involved in leading risk management investi-gations need an in-depth understanding of the NPSA root-cause analysis methodology. A typical risk management team for a maternity unit might consist of a senior obstetrician, a training grade doctor, a midwife, an anaesthetist, a neonatologist and the unit manager.[5] Moreover, it is important to accept that risk management is a process relevant to all stakeholders in the organisation.

Future research

Risk management seems like an excellent idea in principle and early reports are encouraging. Currently, there is a relative paucity of literature regarding monitoring and preventing obstetric adverse events. The NHSLA has defined three levels of CNST and healthcare trusts that fulfil the requirements for each can earn up to 30% discount on their insurance, as they are thought to be practising more safely and therefore reducing their litigation costs. However there has been no proven correlation between CNST level and obstetric claims.[25]

Training has been at the forefront of many enquiries in relation to reducing risk, and obstetric training has been shown to improve patient outcomes.[18,25]

The Adverse Outcomes Index (AOI) is a set of ten quality indicators (obtained using a Delphi process) and interventions such as expert reviews, protocol standardisation, training in team skills and electronic fetal monitoring interpretation have been shown to significantly reduce the AOI.[26]

More research is needed to look at whether risk management inter-ventions actually make a difference to patient outcomes. It would not be possible to conduct a randomised controlled trial (which would be the 'gold standard') on a specific intervention, as this would require suspending all other quality improvement measures during this time, which would be unethical and impracticable. Research should be aimed at developing tools, effective interventions and automation of dashboard technologies using standard datasets. These tools should be generalisable and easily available to all risk management teams.

References

1. Neilsen PE, Goldman MB, Mann S, Shapiro DE, Marcus RG, Pratt SD, et al. Effects of teamwork training on adverse outcomes and process of care in labor and delivery: a randomised controlled trial. *Obstet Gynecol* 2007;109:48–55.

2. Joint Commission. Preventing Infant Death and Injury During Delivery. Sentinel Event Alert Issue 30; 21 July 2004 [http://www.jointcommission.org/SentinelEvents/SentinelEventAlert/sea_30.htm].

3. Lewis G, editor. Saving Mothers' Lives: Reviewing Maternal Deaths to Make Motherhood Safer 2003–2005. The Seventh Report of the Confidential Enquiries into Maternal Deaths in the United Kingdom. London: CEMACH; 2007 [http://www.cmace.org.uk/getdoc/319fb647-d2c6-4b47-b6a0-a853a2f4de1b/Maternal-1.aspx].

4. NHS Litigation Authority. Claims. Factsheet 5 2008/09 [http://www.nhsla.com/claims].

5. Royal College of Obstetricians and Gynaecologists. *Improving Patient Safety: Risk Management for Maternity and Gynaecology*. Clinical Governance Advice No. 2. London: RCOG Press: 2009 [http://www.rcog.org.uk/improving-patient-safety-risk-management-maternity-and-gynaecology].

6. Healthcare Commission. Investigation into 10 Maternal Deaths at, or Following Delivery at, Northwick Park Hospital, North West London Hospital NHS Trust, Between April 2002 and April 2005. London: Commission for Healthcare Audit and Inspection; 2006 [http://www.cqc.org.uk/_db/_documents/Northwick_tagged.pdf].

7. Sibanda T, Sibanda N, Siasskos D, Sivananthan S, Robinson Z, Winter C, *et al.* Prospective evaluation of a continuous monitoring and quality-improvement system for reducing adverse neonatal outcomes. *Am J Obstet Gynecol* 2009;201:480.e1–6.

8. Department of Health. *Maternity Matters: Choice, Access and Continuity of Care in a Safe Service*. London: DH; 2008 [http://www.dh.gov.uk/en/Publicationsand statistics/Publications/PublicationsPolicyAndGuidance/DH_073312].

9. Kingdon C, Neilson J, Singleton V, Gyte G, Hart A, Gabbay M, et al. Choice and birth method: mixed-method study of caesarean delivery for maternal request. *BJOG* 2009;116:886–95.

10. Kings Fund. Safe Births: Everybody's Business: An Independent Inquiry into the Safety of Maternity services in England. London: King's Fund; 2008 [http://www.kingsfund.org.uk/publications/safe_births.html].

11. Royal College of Obstetricians and Gynaecologists, Royal College of Anaesthetists, Royal College of Midwives and Royal College of Paediatrics and Child Health. *Safer Childbirth: Minimum Standards for the Organisation and Delivery of Care in Labour*. London; RCOG Press; 2007 [http://www.rcog.org.uk/

womens-health/clinical-guidance/safer-childbirth-minimum-standards-organisation-and-delivery-care-la].

12. National Childbirth Trust. NCT Document Summary: Towards Better Births: A review of maternity services in England. 2008 [http://www.nctpregnancyand babycare.com/ about-us/what-we-do/policy/keystakeholder-england].

13. Royal College of Anaesthetists, Royal College of Midwives, Royal College of Obstetricians and Gynaecologists, Royal College of Paediatrics and Child Health. *Standards for Maternity Care. Report of a Working Party*. London: RCOG Press; 2008 [http://www.rcog.org.uk/womens-health/clinical-guidance/standards-maternity-care].

14. Royal College of Obstetricians and Gynaecologists. *Maternity Dashboard: Clinical Performance and Governance Scorecard*. Good Practice No 7. London: RCOG; 2008 [http://www.rcog.org.uk/womens-health/clinical-guidance/maternity-dashboard-clinical-performance-and-governance-score-card].

15. Sibanda T, Sibanda N. The CUSUM chart method as a tool for continuous monitoring of clinical outcomes using routinely collected data. *BMC Med Res Methodol* 2007;7:46. DOI:10.1186/1471-2288-7-46.

16. Draycott T, Sibanda T, Owen L, Akande V, Winter C, Reading S, et al. Does training in obstetric emergencies improve neonatal outcome? *BJOG* 2006;113:177–82.

17. Reason J. Human error: models and management. *BMJ* 2000;320:768–70.

18. Reason J. *Human error*. New York: Cambridge University Press; 1990.

19. Healthcare Commission. *Towards Better Births. A Review of Maternity Services in England*. London: Commission for Healthcare Audit and Inspection; 2008 [http://www.cqc.org.uk/publications.cfm?fde_id=625].

20. Black RS, Brocklehurst P. A systemic review of training in acute obstetric emergencies. *BJOG* 2003;110:837–41.

21. Draycott T, Crofts JF, Ash JP, Wilson LV, Yard E, Sibanda T, et al. Improving neonatal outcome through practical shoulder dystocia training. *Obstet Gynecol* 2008;112:14–20.

22. MacKenzie IZ, Shah M, Lean K, Dutton S, Newdick H, Tucker DE. Management of shoulder dystocia: trends in incidence and maternal and neonatal morbidity. *Obstet Gynecol* 2007;110:1059–68.

23. Kirkpatrick D. *Evaluating Training Programs: The Four Levels*. 2nd ed. San Francisco: Berrett-Kochler Publishers; 1998.

24. Siassakos D, Crofts J, Winter C, Weiner C, Draycott T. The active components of effective training in obstetric emergencies. *BJOG* 2009;116:1028–32.

25. Collins, K, Barnfield S, Scholefield H, Draycott T. Is there a correlation between trust maternity claims and CNST level? Poster presented at the British Congress of Obstetrics and Gynaecology, London, 2007.

26. Pettker CM, Thung SF, Norwitz ER, Buhimschi CS, Raab CA, Copel JA, et al. Impact of a comprehensive patient strategy on obstetric adverse events. *Am J Obstet Gynecol* 2009;200:492.e1–8.

CHAPTER 15
Place of birth

Leroy Edozien and Heather Mellows

Key points

✓ Genuine choice depends on the woman and her partner having adequate and appropriate evidence-based information, given at the correct time, to support their decision making.
✓ Providers and commissioners should ensure that appropriate clinical governance, including staffing levels and reliable processes for transfer to obstetric care where necessary, are in place, with due attention given to achieving a balance between choice and safety.

Introduction

Providers of maternity care have a responsibility to assist the woman and her partner in making an informed choice of place of birth. The options include the home, a midwifery-led maternity unit (which may be free-standing or adjacent to a hospital unit) or a consultant-led hospital delivery suite (Box 15.1). The problem with making an informed choice is that robust information required for making this choice is not available. Furthermore, transitions between risk levels could be swift and unpredictable.

Concentrating on the place of birth perhaps detracts from the importance of enshrining the appropriate philosophy of care. Every woman needs a midwife; some need doctors too.[1] Care should be seamless and family-centred so that the woman and her birth partner are in partnership with the healthcare professionals.

Background

Place of birth (Box 15.1) has been a matter of debate for half a century. Until the latter part of the 20th century there was little choice in place of birth and the majority of women delivered at home. The tide began to turn following the publication of the 1946 survey of maternity care in Britain, a report that asserted that 'until the incidence of [obstetric] emergencies can be reduced, there is a good case for the encouragement of institutional delivery'.[2] Subsequently, the proportion of hospital confinements progressively increased and this trend was reinforced by the publication in 1970 of the Peel report, which strongly recommended that 'the resources of modern medicine should be available to all mothers, [and] sufficient facilities should be provided to allow for 100% hospital deliveries'.[3]

Box 15.1 Options for the place of birth

- Home birth, supported by a midwife
- Birth in a local midwifery facility or birth centre
  - based in the community (free standing)

    or
  - based in a hospital (independent of, but adjacent to, an obstetric unit)
- Hospital birth supported by a maternity team, including obstetricians and midwives, consultant-led (obstetric) unit

The Peel report emphasised the need for close links between hospital and health centres and recommended that 'medical and midwifery care should be provided by consultants, general practitioners and midwives working as teams'. It also recommended that 'small isolated obstetric units should be replaced by larger combined consultant and general practitioner units in general hospitals. In the latter units all beds and facilities should be shared'.

The shift from home to hospital birth promoted by Peel was endorsed by an expert committee report in 1984,[4] which bears remarkable resemblance to the modern policy outlined in the National Service Framework (NSF) for Children, Young People and Maternity, emphasising the health and safety of the mother, her experience, choice, need for information and preparation for parenthood and the need to make fathers welcome.[5]

Twenty-two years after the Peel report, 99% of births took place in (hospital) maternity units. However, a sharp rise in interventionist care occurred in tandem with the dominance of hospital births. Rates of episiotomy, caesarean section and, most controversially, 'social' induction of labour rose sharply. A foreseeable backlash ensued. The

House of Commons Health Select Committee challenged the 1984 guidance that 'every mother should be encouraged to have her baby in a maternity unit where emergency facilities are available'. The Committee said it 'had to draw the conclusion that the policy of encouraging all women to give birth in hospital cannot be justified on the grounds of safety'.[6] As a result, the Government set up the Expert Maternity Group whose report, *Changing Childbirth*, aimed to place women at the centre of their care.[7] This report envisaged that, within 5 years, at least 30% of women delivered in a maternity unit would be admitted under the management of a midwife. However, this recommendation has not yet materialised.

With the acknowledgement that healthy mothers have healthy babies that grow into healthy adults, maternity services were included in the NSF for Children, Young People and Maternity.[5] This is a comprehensive framework for provision of maternity care, covering the whole pathway from prepregnancy through to the transition to parenthood: a policy that is seen to be all-encompassing and appropriate for fulfilling the vision that 'women have easy access to supportive, high quality maternity services, designed around their individual needs and those of their babies'.[7]

What women want

Women want safe delivery but they also want to be in control and to be able to make informed decisions. A poll conducted as part of the *Changing Childbirth* work reported that, while 98% of women gave birth in a consultant unit, 72% would have at least liked the option of a different system of care and delivery and, of those, 22% would have liked the choice of home birth and 44% a midwife-led domino (Domiciliary IN and Out) delivery. It was noted that whether the mother was putting herself and her baby at greater risk by choosing to have her baby away from a hospital setting was uncertain, but it was also suggested that professionals cannot quantify the enriching experience that some women feel when they have their baby in a place of their choice. The need for real choice based on clear, unbiased advice was considered paramount.

In the more recent Healthcare Commission Survey, most women in England reported being given the choice of where to have their baby (median trust reported 80%).[8] Fifty-seven percent were offered home birth and 51% of women given the choice of where to have their baby said they had been provided with enough information by midwives or doctors to help them decide. This suggests that most women opt for delivery in a midwifery or obstetric unit despite having the option of delivery at home. In a study conducted in Scotland, most rural women expressed a preference to give birth in hospital because they felt safer.[9] In the National Sentinel Caesarean Section Audit, more than 90% of mothers expressed a wish to have a birth that was the safest option for their baby.[10] Their own safety, a desire for a quick recovery and a birth that would not impede breastfeeding were also strong preferences.

Safety concerns

While there is no consensus regarding the safety of home births,[11–14] it is agreed that the best available data are poor and that 'advice has been based on the absence of evidence of adverse outcomes, rather than on evidence of absence of adverse outcomes'.[14] There are a number of reasons why there are no robust data to inform women on the safety of home births. These include:

- Women opting for home births are more likely to be in a higher socio-economic class, have higher levels of education and be in employment: factors that positively influence perinatal outcome.
- Prior selection of 'high-risk' cases for hospital confinement is a confounding factor, as is inclusion of women with high-risk pregnancies in home birth safety statistics, so comparisons have to be limited to well-defined low-risk groups.
- Outcomes are different for planned and unplanned home births.
- Policies and practices regarding transfer of labouring women from home to hospital may vary from one area to another.
- Choice of place of birth is not always documented at booking. Even when this is recorded, complications developing later in pregnancy mean that some women shift from low to high risk between booking and delivery.
- Data on perinatal mortality attributable solely or primarily to intrapartum factors are not routinely collected. As perinatal mortality among women at low risk is low, large numbers of women are required for a study to be able to draw clinically meaningful conclusions.

These factors could be addressed in a random-allocation study, but women are not keen to be 'randomised' to a place of birth.[15] Factual information will become available from the Birthplace study, which aims 'to provide evidence about important childbirth outcomes that women and health professionals can use to support and inform the choices and decisions that are made when planning the place of birth'.[16]

Risk assessment, workforce, cost and other factors

Policy considerations regarding place of birth must look beyond studies of perinatal mortality; issues such as selection of women, staffing and cost are also important. Unless future evidence dictates otherwise, home birth is an option that should be open to appropriately selected women who are at low risk of obstetric complications and at low risk of being transferred to hospital having laboured at home. The challenge is to correctly categorise such women. It is clear that a woman's own circumstances may dictate that birth in a hospital with facilities to manage all eventualities may be the safest option for her.

Capacity constraints – particularly workforce issues – may inhibit choice. It is usual practice for two midwives to attend a home birth, although in some services maternity support workers are being trained to assist the midwife. It is also sometimes the case that, where a service is under pressure, home birth is restricted so as to retain midwives within the hospital unit.

Financial pressures in the NHS will be increasingly influential in forging the direction of care delivery. As far as we are aware, no economic modelling has been undertaken to compare the costs of birth in different settings and across risk strata in contemporary practice.

Service modelling and care pathways

Unpublished customer insight research, commissioned by the Department of Health, clarified the decision journey for women in choosing location of birth. Women often felt that they had to make the decision too early, sometimes at booking, when they had barely had time to get used to the fact that they were pregnant, let alone know where they would be most comfortable giving birth.

Figure 15.1 gives a schematic representation of the ideal decision making pathway through pregnancy. What is important is that women and their partners understand the principles behind risk assessment and the implications of the choices they make. The three elements of quality laid out by Lord Darzi in the *Next Stage Review* (safety, effectiveness and patient satisfaction) are exemplified in the decisions surrounding place of birth.[17]

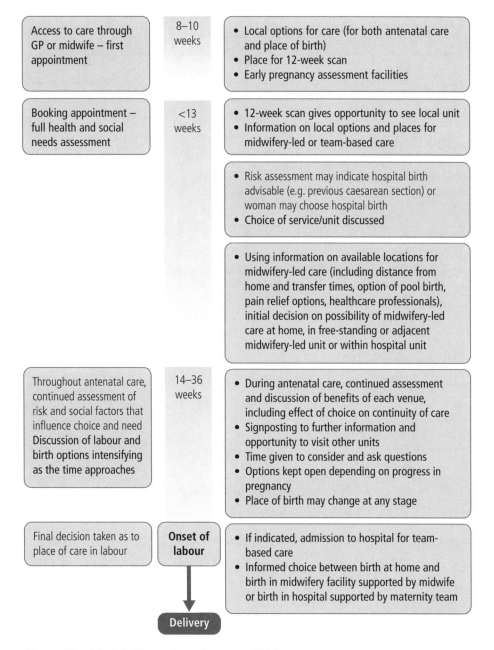

| | 8–10 weeks | • Local options for care (for both antenatal care and place of birth)
• Place for 12-week scan
• Early pregnancy assessment facilities |

Access to care through GP or midwife – first appointment

Booking appointment – full health and social needs assessment — <13 weeks
• 12-week scan gives opportunity to see local unit
• Information on local options and places for midwifery-led or team-based care

• Risk assessment may indicate hospital birth advisable (e.g. previous caesarean section) or woman may choose hospital birth
• Choice of service/unit discussed

• Using information on available locations for midwifery-led care (including distance from home and transfer times, option of pool birth, pain relief options, healthcare professionals), initial decision on possibility of midwifery-led care at home, in free-standing or adjacent midwifery-led unit or within hospital unit

Throughout antenatal care, continued assessment of risk and social factors that influence choice and need Discussion of labour and birth options intensifying as the time approaches — 14–36 weeks
• During antenatal care, continued assessment and discussion of benefits of each venue, including effect of choice on continuity of care
• Signposting to further information and opportunity to visit other units
• Time given to consider and ask questions
• Options kept open depending on progress in pregnancy
• Place of birth may change at any stage

Final decision taken as to place of care in labour — **Onset of labour**
• If indicated, admission to hospital for team-based care
• Informed choice between birth at home and birth in midwifery facility supported by midwife or birth in hospital supported by maternity team

Delivery

Figure 15.1 Ideal decision pathway for place of birth

Figure 15.2 shows a suggested algorithm of possible alternatives following risk and needs assessment at booking that can inform the initial and subsequent choice regarding place of birth.

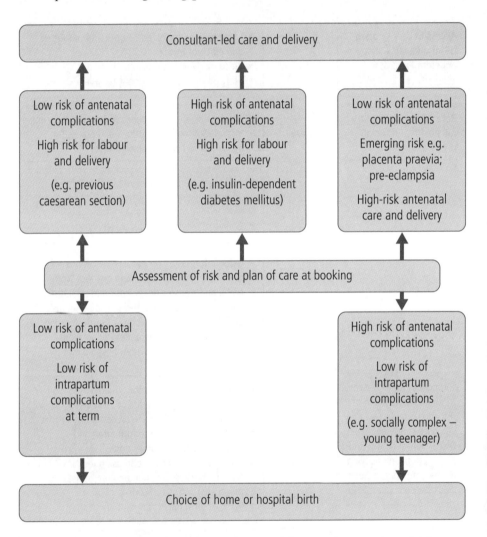

Figure 15.2 Assessment of needs and risk and how it influences choice in place of delivery

The use of maternity standards to inform choice and decisions in place of birth

The *Standards for Maternity Care* cover the whole pregnancy pathway.[18] Several standards relate to the preparation for the woman and her partner to inform decisions on place of birth.

Standard 1 allows for prepregnancy counselling so that women may be made aware of the options when they become pregnant. Standard 2 provides for women with pre-existing conditions to have prepregnancy counselling to ensure they are aware of the implications of their history or condition on choice of place of care and birth.

Standards 3 and 5 ensure that women know how to access care so that there is time for full assessment of their needs and choices and for information sharing, which enables them to make appropriate choices during the development of their plan of care.

Standards 6, 7 and 8 set out the requirements of women with pre-existing medical and social conditions as well as pre-existing and developing mental health conditions in pregnancy and define the need for multidisciplinary care.

Standards 10 and 11 emphasise the fact that a woman's clinical and other needs may change during pregnancy and this would include needs relating to place of birth. At any stage a woman may need referral for multidisciplinary care. Standard 12 summarises the standards defined in *Safer Childbirth* required for intrapartum care in every setting and location.[19] Standard 13 defines the needs of the baby.

Conclusion

Deciding on place of birth is just one of the choices that a woman and her partner need to make in their journey to parenthood. Genuine choice depends on the woman and her partner having adequate and appropriate information, given at the correct time, to support their decision making. Care providers must have the knowledge and ability to present the risks and benefits in a manner that the woman and her partner can understand so that trust is developed and maintained throughout pregnancy and the birth. Robust statistics on safety are not yet available but use of the published *Maternity Standards* will facilitate tailored information-giving and enable evidence-based decisions.[18]

Providers and commissioners should ensure that appropriate clinical governance, including adequate midwifery staffing levels and reliable processes for transfer to obstetric care where necessary, is in place with due attention given to achieving a balance between choice and safety. The importance of this balance is illustrated by a meta-analysis that showed that, when compared with conventional institutional settings, home-like institutional birth settings reduce the likelihood of medical interventions, increase maternal satisfaction, rates of normal birth and breastfeeding and reduce the likelihood of episiotomy, but are associated with a trend towards higher perinatal mortality.[20]

Commissioners should be aware of local factors (such as geography, workforce and resources) that determine the availability of options and should monitor statistics such as rates and times of transfer of labouring women from home to hospital. As well as ensuring availability of different birth settings, commissioners should obtain assurances that each birth setting enshrines a philosophy of care that promotes normal birth and pursues not only good clinical outcomes but also good psychological outcomes.[21]

References

1. Department of Health. *Making it Better: For Mother and Baby: Clinical Case for Change*. Report by Sheila Shribman. National Clinical Director for Children, Young People and Maternity Services. London; DH; 2007 [http://www.dh.gov.uk/en/Publicationsandstatistics/Publications/ PublicationsPolicyAndGuidance/DH_065053]
2. Royal College of Obstetricians and Gynaecologists; Population Investigation Committee. Maternity in Great Britain. Survey Undertaken by a Joint Committee of the Royal College of Obstetricians and Gynaecologists and the Population Investigation Committee. Oxford; Oxford University Press; 1946.
3. Standing Maternity and Midwifery Advisory Committee. *Domiciliary Midwifery and Maternity Bed Needs: Report of a Sub-committee*. London; HMSO; 1970.
4. Maternity Services Advisory Committee. Maternity Care in Action. First Report of the Maternity Services Advisory Committee Part II: Care During Childbirth (Intrapartum c): A Guide to Good Practice and a Plan for Action. London: HMSO; 1985.
5. Department of Health. *National Service Framework for Children, Young People and Maternity Services Standard 11: Maternity Services*. London: DH; 2004 [http://www.dh.gov.uk/en/Publicationsandstatistics/Publications/PublicationsPolicy AndGuidance/Browsable/DH_4094336].
6. House of Commons. Health Select Committee. *Second Report, Session 1991–1992: Maternity Services*. HMSO; 1992.
7. Department of Health. Changing Childbirth. Part I: Report of the Expert Maternity Group. London: HMSO; 1993.

8. Healthcare Commission. *Towards Better Births. A Review of Maternity Services in England*. London: Commission for Healthcare Audit and Inspection; 2008 [http://www.cqc.org.uk/publications.cfm?fde_id=625].
9. Pitchforth E, Watson V, Tucker J, Ryan M, van Teijlingen E, Farmer J, et al. Models of intrapartum care and women's trade-offs in remote and rural Scotland: a mixed-methods study. *BJOG* 2008;115:560–9.
10. Royal College of Obstetricians and Gynaecologists Clinical Effectiveness Support Unit. *The National Sentinel Caesarean Section Audit Report*. London; RCOG Press; 2001.
11. Mori R, Dougherty M, Whittle M. An estimation of intrapartum-related perinatal mortality rates for booked home births in England and Wales between 1994 and 2003. *BJOG* 2008;115:554–9.
12. Wiegers TA, Kierse MJ, vabn der Bergs GA. Outcome of planned home and planned hospital births in low risk pregnancies: prospective study in midwifery practices in The Netherlands. *BMJ* 1996;313:1309–13.
13. Gyte G, Dodwell M, Newburn M, Sandall J, Macfarlane A, Bewley S. Estimating intrapartum-related Perinatal mortality rates for booked home births: when the best available data are not good enough. *BJOG* 2009;116:933–42.
14. Van Weel C, van der Velden K, Largo-Jannssen T. Home births revisited: the continuing search for better evidence. *BJOG* 2009;116:1149–50.
15. Hendrix M, Van Horck M, Moreta D, Neiman F, Nieuwenhuijze M, Severns J, et al. Why women do not accept randomisation for place of birth: feasibility of a RCT in the Netherlands. *BJOG* 2009;116:537–44.
16. National Perinatal Epidemiology Unit. The Birthplace in England Research Programme [http://www.npeu.ox.ac.uk/birthplace].
17. Department of Health. *High Quality Care for All: NHS Next Stage Review Final Report*. Cm7432. London: The Stationery Office; 2008 [http://www.dh.gov.uk/en/publicationsandstatistics/publications/publicationspolicyandguidance/DH_085825].
18. Royal College of Anaesthetists, Royal College of Midwives, Royal College of Obstetricians and Gynaecologists, Royal College of Paediatrics and Child Health. *Standards for Maternity Care. Report of a Working Party*. London: RCOG Press; 2008 [http://www.rcog.org.uk/womens-health/clinical-guidance/standards-maternity-care].
19. Royal College of Obstetricians and Gynaecologists, Royal College of Anaesthetists, Royal College of Midwives and Royal College of Paediatrics and Child Health. *Safer Childbirth: Minimum Standards for the Organisation and Delivery of Care in Labour*. London; RCOG Press; 2007 [http://www.rcog.org.uk/womens-health/clinical-guidance/safer-childbirth-minimum-standards-organisation-and-delivery-care-la].
20. Hodnett ED, Downe S, Edwards N, Walsh D. Home-like versus conventional institutional settings for birth. *Cochrane Database Syst Rev* 2005;(1):CD000012. DOI: 10.1002/14651858.CD000012.pub2.
21. Department of Health. *Maternity Matters: Choice, Access and Continuity of Care in a Safe Service*. London: DH; 2008 [http://www.dh.gov.uk/en/Publicationsandstatistics/Publications/PublicationsPolicyAndGuidance/DH_073312].

CHAPTER 16

High-risk pregnancy and neonatal services

Cornelia Hagmann and Jane Hawdon

Key points

✓ A written and agreed postnatal plan should be outlined before birth; for example, parents should be advised that delivery should occur at a unit that can provide the appropriate level of neonatal care for anticipated gestation, birth weight and any neonatal complications.

✓ Mothers and babies should remain together unless there is a clear clinical indication for admission for enhanced care. The care of the baby must not be inappropriately invasive.

✓ Transitional care, where babies remain with their mother but may be monitored closely, is the ideal setting for babies in these circumstances.

■ Introduction

Understanding of the occurrence and severity of likely neonatal complications is important when planning antenatal care and birth, and in counselling parents. As far as possible, a written and agreed postnatal plan should be outlined before birth; for example, parents should be advised that delivery should occur at a unit that can provide the appropriate level of neonatal care for anticipated gestation, birth weight and any neonatal complications. They should also be advised of the likely length of stay for the baby. Risks must not be overestimated, especially when control of maternal condition is good. Mothers and babies should remain together unless there is a clear clinical indication for admission for enhanced care. The care of the baby must not be inappropriately invasive. Transitional care, where babies remain with their mother but may be monitored closely, is the ideal setting for many babies if circumstances permit.

The only contraindications to babies receiving their mothers' breast milk are maternal HIV infection, maternal cytotoxic medication, mater-nal radioisotope administration and heavy or chaotic illicit drug use. For all other conditions discussed below, the advantages of the baby receiving mother's breast milk are even greater than in the general population.

Neonatal complications of high-risk pregnancy

Diabetes during pregnancy

There is an increased incidence of congenital abnormalities, macrosomia, birth injuries, hypoxia–ischaemia, polycythaemia, hyperbilirubinaemia, hypomagnesiaemia, hypoglycaemia, hypocalcaemia and cardiomyopathy in babies of mothers with diabetes.[1-3]

Babies of women with diabetes should remain with their mothers unless there is a clinical complication or there are abnormal clinical signs that warrant admission for intensive or special care. There should be support for early breastfeeding. Blood glucose monitoring should com-mence at 2–4 hours after birth and testing for other complications should be considered if there are abnormal clinical signs.[4]

Hypertensive disorder during pregnancy and pre-eclampsia

Hypertension in pregnancy and pre-eclampsia are associated with fetal growth restriction (FGR), prematurity and low Apgar scores at birth.[5] Most neonatal complications are consequent upon the gestational age at birth or degree of FGR.[6]

If the baby is growth-restricted or if the mother is treated with a beta-blocker, blood glucose monitoring is indicated; even if the baby is born at term, early discharge should be avoided.[6]

Autoimmune disorders

Systemic lupus erythematosus

Preterm birth is increased in pregnant women with systemic lupus erythe-matosus (SLE)[7-9] and has been related to a history of fetal loss, hypertension and use of prednisolone at a dose of 20 mg/day higher.[8] Neonatal complications include FGR, congenital heart block and neonatal lupus. Predictors for FGR are low levels of C3 and C4, hypertension and absence of anti-SSA/Ro antibodies.[8,10] Congenital heart block and neonatal lupus are associated with maternal anti-SSA antibodies pregnancies.[7,11] Such infants with congenital heart block are usually asymptomatic.

If FGR is present, close monitoring of blood glucose level and early feeding should be initiated. If there is concern about the baby's heart rate, referral for cardiology opinion is indicated.

Myasthenia gravis

Transplacental transmission of acetylcholine receptor (AchR) antibodies can lead to neonatal myasthenia gravis, which affects 10–20% of babies born to mothers with the condition.[12] Fetal distress can be the first sign of a pre-existing neurological condition.[13,14] Neonatal myasthenia gravis can present with transient respiratory problems and difficulties in feeding and swallowing.[12] In rare cases, arthrogryposis multiplex congenita can be caused.[15]

Babies need to be monitored closely during the first couple of days after delivery for signs of respiratory distress and muscle weakness as the symptoms of neonatal myasthenia gravis usually occur 12–48 hours after birth.[16] If clinically indicated, admit the baby to the neonatal unit.

Idiopathic alloimmune thrombocytopenia

Thrombocytopenia occurs in about 10% of newborn babies whose mothers have autoantibodies and the incidence of intracranial haemorrhage is 1% or less.[17,18] A platelet count on cord blood or by peripheral blood sampling should be carried out soon after birth. In newborn babies with normal platelet counts (greater than $150 \times 10^9/l$) no further tests are necessary. If thrombocytopenia is present, repeat a platelet count after 2–3 days, as platelet counts are often at their lowest at this time before rising spontaneously by day 7 in most cases.[19] Babies with thrombocytopenia should have a cranial ultrasound scan to monitor for intraventricular haemorrhage.

Thyroid conditions during pregnancy

Maternal hypothyroidism

Combined maternal and fetal hypothyroidism is associated with abnormal neurodevelopmental outcome. The most severely affected babies have mental restriction and motor impairment. Altered neuropsychological development (decreased IQ) has been reported in offspring of mothers with thyroid underfunction, even when maternal disease is mild and considered subclinical.[20,21] Early clinical signs at and after birth include large posterior fontanelle, umbilical hernia, goitre, feeding difficulties, prolonged jaundice, lethargy, respiratory problems and abdominal distension.

Neonatal thyroid-stimulating hormone (TSH) screening is performed in the UK by blood sampling between days 5 and 10. The diagnosis is confirmed if high TSH and low free T_4 (thyroxine) are present. Prompt treatment with thyroxine should be commenced and regular growth, clinical and biochemical assessments are mandatory. Babies of mothers with autoimmune thyroiditis require measurement of thyroid antibodies.

Maternal hyperthyroidism

TSH receptor-stimulating antibodies can cross the placenta and produce fetal and neonatal thyrotoxicosis. Clinical symptoms of babies include palpable goitre, irritability, restlessness, jitteriness, tachycardia, arrhythmias, excessive appetite with inadequate weight gain, sweating, flushing, hepatosplenomegaly, jaundice and accelerated bone maturation. An increased mortality rate is reported.[22]

The baby should be assessed clinically for signs of thyrotoxicosis. If necessary, treatment with antithyroid medication should be started and the thyroid function assessed regularly. Neonatal thyrotoxicosis usually resolves after 2–5 months and withdrawal of antithyroid medication should be initiated at that time.

Maternal epilepsy during pregnancy

Babies of mothers with epilepsy have a two- to three-fold higher risk of congenital malformations, mainly associated with antiepileptic drugs.[23,24] Malformations include spina bifida, cleft lip and palate and cardiac malformations.[24–26] There is an increased risk of vitamin K deficiency in the newborn of mothers who take anticonvulsants during pregnancy.[27] A detailed clinical examination of the baby should be undertaken to detect any malformation. Cardiac echocardiography should be performed and intramuscular vitamin K given to the newborn.

■ Heart disease during pregnancy

The prevalence of congenital heart disease (CHD) in babies born to mothers with heart disease is 3.1% compared with 1.3% in the general population.[28] The recurrence risk varies according to the parent's condition: from 3% in tetralogy of Fallot to 10% for atrial septal defect,[29] 10% for coarctation of the aorta[30] and 15.6% for ventricular septal defect.[31]

A clinical examination of the baby should be undertaken, including four-limb blood pressure. Echocardiography should be performed before discharge, unless there has been a reassuring antenatal scan by a specialist in fetal echocardiography.

■ Mental health concerns during pregnancy

Maternal anxiety disorders, such as panic disorder, obsessive–compulsive disorder, post-traumatic stress disorder, social anxiety disorders or phobias during pregnancy, are associated with an increased risk of spontaneous miscarriage,[32] preterm birth[33] and delivery complications.[34] Women with schizophrenia are at higher risk of stillbirth, infant death, preterm delivery, low birth weight, small-for-gestational-age infants and an increased rate of fetal malformations.[35,36]

Clinical management of psychiatric illness during pregnancy and lactation encompasses an assessment of the risk of exposure of the mother and neonate to medication during pregnancy. A multidisciplinary team review should be undertaken to address any safeguarding issues.[37]

■ Illicit drug use during pregnancy

Illicit drug use during pregnancy can significantly increase perinatal morbidity, low birth weight, a small head and preterm birth.[38–40] Sexually transmitted diseases and hepatitis are more common in substance abusers; hence, these babies are at increased risk of vertical transmission of infections. Babies of substance abusers may develop neonatal abstinence syndrome requiring treatment and admission to a neonatal unit. Initial signs of withdrawal are central nervous disturbances such as rhythmic tremulousness, excessive alertness, agitation, activity with frantic sucking of fingers and hands and hypertonus. Disorganised coordination of sucking and swallowing, vomiting and regurgitation are common. Seizures can also occur. These babies need to be monitored for signs of withdrawal and an analysis of urine and/or meconium should be requested if the nature of the exposure is not clear from maternal testing.

Breastfeeding is usually not recommended for mothers using heroin. However, in mothers on methadone, morphine or codeine, breast-feeding is not contraindicated if the mother is stable and no polydrug abuse is present.

Maternal infection

Maternal viral infection, such as hepatitis B, hepatitis C and HIV, is rarely associated with neonatal complications. However, other maternal infections such as rubella, cytomegalovirus, varicella and toxoplasmosis can transmit to the fetus and cause congenital abnormalities or infection, depending on the stage of gestation.

Maternal bacterial infection may be associated with poor condition at birth and neonatal bacteraemia or meningitis with a risk of long-term neurological sequelae or even death. The relationship between maternal and fetal cytokines secondary to perinatal infection and brain injury is the subject of debate and ongoing research. Maternal tuberculosis rarely carries a risk of transmission to the fetus through bacteraemic spread but there is a significant risk of neonatal transmission.

Babies born to mothers with HIV infection, high-infectivity hepatitis B and tuberculosis require prophylactic treatment. Babies with proven neonatal infection require immediate treatment. If congenital viral infection is suspected, investigation for associated abnormalities should be undertaken. In all newborn babies, risk factors for bacterial infection should be considered.

Concerns regarding safeguarding

Babies are at risk of harm and neglect, even in the early neonatal period, if there are sufficient concerns regarding maternal or paternal mental health, drug use, personality disorder or learning disability. Therefore, all women should have a risk assessment, including enquiry into the wellbeing of other children. Where there is concern, there should be an agreed multidisciplinary care plan for the mother before birth and for the mother and baby after birth. The baby should not be discharged until clear and secure arrangements are in place for their wellbeing.

■ References

1. Jones CW. Gestational diabetes and its impact on the neonate. *Neonatal Netw* 2001;20:17–23.
2. Esakoff TF, Cheng YW, Sparks TN, Caughey AB The association between birthweight 4000g or greater and Perinatal outcomes in patients with and without gestational diabetes mellitus. *Am J Obstet Gynecol* 2009;200:672.el–4.
3. Jensen DM, Sørensen B, Feilberg-Jørgensen N, Westergaard JG, Beck-Nielsen H. Maternal and Perinatal outcomes in 143 Danish women with gestational diabetes mellitus and 143 controls with a similar risk profile. *Diabet Med* 2000;17:281–6.
4. National Institute for Health and Clinical Excellence. *Diabetes in Pregnancy: Management of Diabetes and its Complications from Preconception to the Postnatal Period*. London: NICE; 2008 [http://guidance.nice.org.uk/CG63].
5. Yücesoy G, Ozkan S, Bodur H, Tan T, Cali kan E, Vural B, *et al*. Maternal and perinatal outcome in pregnancies complicated with hypertensive disorder of pregnancy: a seven year experience of a tertiary care center. *Arch Gynecol Obstet* 2005;273:43–9.
6. Teh CL, Wong JS, Ngeh NK, Loh WL. Systemic lupus erythematosus pregnancies: a case series from a tertiary, East Malyasian hospital. *Lupus* 2009;18:278–82.
7. Le Thi Huong D, Wechsler B, Piette JC, Bletry O, Godeau P. Pregnancy and its outcome in systemic lupus erythematosus. *QJM* 1994;87:721–9.
8. Cavallasca JA, Laborde HA, Ruda-Vega H, Nasswetter GG. Maternal and fetal outcomes of 72 pregnancies in Argentine patients with systemic lupus erythematosus (SLE). *Clin Rheumatol* 2008;27:41–6.
9. Ramsey-Goldman R, Hom D, Deng JS, Ziegler GC, Kahl LE, Steen VD, et al. Anti-SS-A antibodies and fetal outcome in maternal systemic lupus erythematosus. *Arthritis Rheum* 1986;29:1269–73.
10. Leu LY, Lan JL. The influence on pregnancy of anti-SSA/Ro antibodies in systemic lupus erythematosus. *Zhonghua Min Guo Wei Sheng Wu Ji Mian Yi Xue Za Zhi* 1992;25:12–20.
11. Brucato A, Doria A, Frassi M, Castellino G, Franceschini F, Faden D, et al. Pregnancy outcome in 100 women with autoimmune diseases and anti-Ro/SSA antibodies: a prospective controlled study. *Lupus* 2002;11:716–21.
12. Papazian, O. Transient neonatal myasthenia gravis. *J Child Neurol* 1992;7:135–41.
13. Hoff JM, Daltveit AK, Gilhus NE. Myasthenia gravis in pregnancy and birth: identifying risk factors, optimising care. *Eur J Neurol* 2007;14:38–43.
14. Adamson SJ, Alessandri LM, Badawi N, Burton PR, Pemberton PJ, Stanley F. Predictors of neonatal encephalopathy in full-term infants. *BMJ* 1995;311:598–602.
15. Vincent A, Newland C, Brueton L, Beeson D, Riemersma S, Huson SM, et al. Arthrogryposis multiplex congenital with maternal autoantibodies specific for a fetal antigen. *Lancet* 1995;346:24–5.
16. Ciafaloni E, Massey JM. The management of myasthenia gravis in pregnancy. *Semin Neurol* 2004;24:95–100.

17. Bussel JB. Immune thrombocytopenia in pregnancy: autoimmune and alloimmue. *J Reprod Immunol* 1997;37:35–61.
18. Bussel JB, Sola-Visner M. Current approaches to the evaluation and management of the fetus and neonate with immune thrombocytopenia. *Semin Perinatol* 2009;33:35–42.
19. Burrows RF, Kelton JG. Low fetal risks in pregnancies associated with idiopathic thrombocytopenic purpura. *Am J Obstet Gynecol* 1990;163:1147–50.
20. Pop VJ, Kuijpens JL, van Baar AL, Verkerk G, van Son MM, de Vijlder JJ, et al. Low maternal free thyroxine concentrations during early pregnancy are associated with impaired psychomotor development in infancy. *Clin Endocrinol (Oxf)* 1999;50:149–55.
21. Haddow JE, Palomaki GE, Allan WC, Williams JR, Knight GJ, Gagnon J, et al. Maternal thyroid deficiency during pregnancy and subsequent neuropsychological development of the child. *N Engl J Med* 1999;341:549–55.
22. Skuza KA, Sills IN, Stene M, Rapaport R. Prediction of neonatal hyperthyroidism in infants born to mothers with Graves disease. *J Pediatr* 1996;128:264–8.
23. Perucca E. Birth defects after prenatal exposure to antiepileptic drugs. *Lancet Neurol* 2005;4:781–6.
24. Veiby G, Daltveit AK, Engelsen BA, Gilhus NE. Pregnancy, delivery, and outcome for the child in maternal epilepsy. *Epilepsia* 2009;50:2130–9.
25. Holmes LB, Baldwin EJ, Smith CR, Habecker E, Glassman L, Wong SL, et al. Increased frequency of isolated cleft palate in infants exposed to lamotrigine during pregnancy. *Neurology* 2008;70:2152–8.
26. Wyszynski DF, Nambisan M, Surve T, Alsdorf RM, Smith CR, Holmes LB; Antiepileptic Drug Pregnancy Registry. Increased rate of major malformations in offspring exposed to valproate during pregnancy. *Neurology* 2005;64:961–5.
27. Moslet U, Hansen ES. A review of vitamin K, epilepsy and pregnancy. *Acta Neurol Scand* 1992;85:39–43.
28. Romano-Zelekha O, Hirsh R, Blieden L, Green M, Shohat T. The risk for congenital heart defects in offspring of individuals with congenital heart defects. *Clin Genet* 2001:59:325–9.
29. Burn J, Brennan P, Little J, Holloway S, Coffey R, Somerville J, et al. Recurrence risks in offspring of adults with major heart defects: results from first cohort of British collaborative study. *Lancet* 1998;351:311–6.
30. Rose V, Gold RJ, Lindsay G, Allen M. A possible increase in the incidence of congenital heart defects among the offspring of affected parents. *J Am Coll Cardiol* 1985;6:376–82.
31. Whittemore R, Wells JA, Castellsague X. A second-generation study of 427 probands with congenital heart defects and their 837 children. *J Am Coll Cardiol* 1994:23:1459–67.
32. Boyles SH, Ness RB, Grisso JA, Markovic N, Bromberger J, CiFelli D. Life event stress and the association with spontaneous abortion in gravid women at an urban emergency department. *Health Psychol* 2000;19:510–4.
33. Berkowitz GS, Kasl SV. The role of psychosocial factors in spontaneous preterm delivery. *J Psychosom Res* 1983:27:283–90.
34. Perkin MR, Bland JM, Peacock JL, Anderson HR. The effect of anxiety and depression during pregnancy on obstetric complications. *Br J Obstet Gynaecol* 1993;100:629–34.
35. Jablensky AV, Morgan V, Zubrick SR, Bower C, Yellachich LA. Pregnancy, delivery, and neonatal complications in a population cohort of women with schizophrenia and major affective disorders. *Am J Psychiatry* 2005;162:79–91.

36. Nyheln A, Ljungberg B, Nilsson-Ehle I. Pharmacokinetics of ceftazidime in febrile neutropenic patients. *Scand J Infect Dis* 2001;33:222–6.
37. Cott AD, Wisner KL. Psychiatric disorders during pregnancy. *Int Rev Psychiatry* 2003:15:217–30.
38. Eyler FD, Behnke M, Conlon M, Woods NS, Wobie K. Birth outcome from a prospective, matched study of prenatal crack/cocaine use: I. Interactive and dose effects on health and growth. *Pediatrics* 1998;101:229–37.
39. Dawkins JL, Tylden E, Colley N, Evans C. Drug abuse in pregnancy: obstetric and neonatal problems. Ten years' experience. *Drug Alcohol Rev* 1997;16:25–31.
40. Chasnoff IJ, Griffith DR, MacGregor S, Dirkes K, Burns KA Temporal patterns of cocaine use in pregnancy. Perinatal outcome. *JAMA* 1989;261:1741–4.

CHAPTER 17

Anaesthesia service provision for maternity services

Vishal Uppal and Elizabeth McGrady

Key points

- ✓ A duty anaesthetist should be immediately available for the delivery suite 24 hours a day.
- ✓ There should be a nominated consultant in charge of obstetric anaesthesia and training.
- ✓ There should be a clear line of communication from the duty anaesthetist to the supervising consultant at all times.
- ✓ When provision of the basic minimum staffing levels is not cost-effective, consideration should be given to amalgamation with other local units.
- ✓ Women should have antenatal access to information about the availability and provision of all types of analgesia and anaesthesia.
- ✓ There should be an agreed system whereby the anaesthetist is given sufficient advance notice of all potential high-risk patients.
- ✓ Separate staffing and resources should be allocated to elective caesarean section lists to prevent delays owing to emergency procedures and provision of regional analgesia in labour.
- ✓ The assistant to the anaesthetist must have no other conflicting duties, must be trained to a recognised national standard and must work regularly in the obstetric unit.
- ✓ The training undertaken by staff in the maternity recovery unit and the facilities must be to the same standard as for general recovery facilities.
- ✓ All grades of anaesthetist who are on-call for the delivery suite but do not have regular sessions there, should spend time in the delivery suite with one of the regular obstetric anaesthesia consultants.
- ✓ Appropriate facilities should be available for the antenatal and peripartum management of the sick obstetric patient.

■ Introduction

This chapter describes the level of service required from anaesthesia departments providing services for obstetric units. In addition to clinical duties, consultant anaesthetists are involved in teaching, training, administration, research and audit.

There should be a dedicated obstetric anaesthesia service for all consultant-led obstetric units as anaesthetists are involved in the care of approximately 60% of pregnant women.[1] This is because of the increasing caesarean section rate in the UK (over 30% in some units), the increasing age of pregnant women and the number of mothers with comorbidities.[2,3] Anaesthesia delay can be a factor in some stillbirths and infant deaths.[4] Concerns have been expressed about the staffing of isolated obstetric units, the level of experience of anaesthesia staff on-call and the reduction of exposure to emergency general anaesthesia in obstetrics.[5,6]

■ What women want

Probably the largest survey of maternal views on analgesia in labour was the 1990 National Birthday Trust Survey of all deliveries in the UK.[7] This survey was carried out over a period of one week and evaluated pain experienced and analgesia provided in labour. It showed that women often underestimated the severity of labour pain: although only 17% of mothers planned to receive an epidural, 24% actually did and 33% planned to use an epidural in a future labour. Comments by the mothers were also reported: several complained that they had not been adequately warned of the severity of labour pain and the consequent need for epidural analgesia, and that epidural analgesia had been delayed or withheld.

While this survey has not been repeated and was conducted nearly 20 years ago, the requirement for an obstetric anaesthesia service must have increased with the continuing rise in the caesarean section rate. It is unlikely that epidural rates have fallen, as comorbidities and obesity have increased.

Most women are unprepared for emergency obstetric anaesthesia, with many receiving information just before the event. After delivery, women often express a preference for earlier information.[8] Women differ in their requirements for antenatal information about regional analgesia and its complications, with some wanting to know every complication, however rare.[9]

National guidance and clinical guidelines

The Obstetric Anaesthetists' Association (OAA) and the Association of Anaesthetists of Great Britain and Ireland (AAGBI) jointly published *Guidelines for Obstetric Anaesthesia Services*.[10] The Royal College of Anaesthetists (RCoA), has published *Guidelines for the Provision of Anaesthetic Services*.[11] The Royal College of Obstetricians and Gynaecologists has produced two relevant guidelines in collaboration with the Royal Colleges of Anaesthetists, Midwives and Paediatrics and Child Health.[12,13] These guidelines aim at developing national standards for maternity care.

The 1997–1999 and 2003–2005 reports of the Confidential Enquiries into Maternal Deaths in the United Kingdom emphasised the need for a dedicated obstetric anaesthesia service for all consultant-led obstetric units, the anaesthetic pre-assessment of women in high-risk categories, early involvement of senior anaesthetists and transfer to units with intensive care facilities for high-risk cases.[5,14]

Service modelling and care pathways

It is important that obstetric anaesthetists develop good working relationships and lines of communication with all other professionals, including those whose care may be needed for difficult pregnancies. This includes midwives and obstetricians, as well as professionals from other disciplines such as intensive care, neurology, cardiology, haematology and other physicians and surgeons. An obstetric anaesthetist should take part in regular multidisciplinary 'labour ward forum' meetings.

A clear line of communication from the duty anaesthetist to the on-call consultant should be assured at all times. The theatre manager should be responsible for maintaining communication with staff groups and ensuring competent staffing and suitable equipping of the theatres. Larger units and those with high caesarean section rates should have elective caesarean section lists with dedicated obstetric, anaesthesia and theatre staff to minimise disruption caused by emergency work.

All obstetric departments should provide and regularly update clinical protocols, which should be readily accessible.[10,11]

Regional analgesia

Most consultant obstetric units should be able to provide regional analgesia on request at all times. Smaller units may be unable to supply dedicated cover at all times, so women booking at such units must be made aware that epidural analgesia may not always be available. Units should have guidelines for the management of epidural blocks and there should be appropriate levels of medical and midwifery staff for delivery of the service.

Emergency caesarean sections

There should be a clear line of communication between the duty anaesthetist, theatre staff and operating departmental personnel/anaesthesia nurse once a decision is made to undertake an emergency caesarean section. The anaesthetist should be informed about the category of urgency of caesarean section.

There should be clear guidelines available for who to call if two emergencies occur simultaneously. Anaesthetists in other parts of the hospital may need to be summoned if the second anaesthetist is attending from home.

▇ Special issues related to service delivery

For the efficient functioning of the obstetric anaesthesia service, the following equipment, support services and facilities are essential. The standards of equipment and monitoring must be the same as those of a non-obstetric anaesthesia service.

Equipment

The delivery suite should be equipped with:

- the facility for rapid bedside estimation of haemoglobin and blood sugar
- monitoring equipment for the measurement of blood pressure, electrocardiogram (ECG), oxygen saturation, temperature and invasive haemodynamic monitoring, if required
- oxygen, suction equipment and access to resuscitation equipment
- active scavenging of waste anaesthetic gas
- a supply of O rhesus-negative blood for emergency use.

Obstetric theatres should be equipped with:

- the standard of monitoring for the conduct of safe anaesthesia for surgery as detailed in the AAGBI guidelines[15]
- a blood warmer allowing the rapid transfusion of blood and fluids and a warm air blower/blankets
- a cell salvage machine for massive blood loss and women who are Jehovah's Witnesses
- a difficult intubation trolley with a variety of laryngoscopes, tracheal tubes, laryngeal masks and other aids for airway management
- an operating table that can safely support a person weighing 160 kg or more
- ultrasound imaging equipment for central vascular access and epidural cannulation for women who are high risk and/or morbidly obese.

Patient-controlled analgesia equipment and infusion devices must be available for postoperative pain relief.

Support services

A system should be in place to ensure that women requiring antenatal referral to the anaesthetist are seen and assessed by a senior anaesthetist within a suitable timeframe, preferably in early pregnancy. There must be adequate secretarial support for the antenatal anaesthesia assessment clinic and other duties of the consultant obstetric anaesthetist, including teaching, research, audit, study, appraisal activities and other administrative work.

Haematology and biochemistry services must be available to provide rapid analysis of blood and other body fluids and to make blood and blood products for transfusion available without delay according to clinical need. Pharmacy services are required for the provision of necessary routine and emergency drugs. Physiotherapy services should be available 24 hours a day for women requiring high-dependency care. There must be rapid availability of radiological services.

Facilities

There should be at least one fully equipped obstetric theatre within the delivery suite readily available for women requiring emergency caesarean section (in addition to one for elective procedures). Adequate recovery room facilities, including the ability to monitor blood pressure, ECG and oxygen saturation, must be available within the delivery suite theatre complex.

A fully equipped high-dependency unit with appropriately trained staff should be available in units caring for high-risk obstetric patients. Access to the intensive care unit must be available for all obstetric patients and preferably available on site. Portable monitoring with the facility for invasive monitoring must be available to facilitate transfer of obstetric patients to the intensive care unit.

For obstetric units on the same site but not actually part of the main hospital, adequate links or transport arrangements must be in place to allow the safe transfer of obstetric patients to the main theatres or intensive care unit.

An anaesthesia office, in proximity to the delivery suite, should be available to the duty anaesthesia team. The room should hold a computer with intra/internet access to facilitate audit of the anaesthesia service and access to up-to-date information. A library of specialist reference books, journals and local multidisciplinary evidence-based guidelines must be available. There should be a separate office available to allow teaching, assessment and appraisal.

Training

Obstetric units with an anaesthesia service should have a nominated consultant responsible for training in obstetric anaesthesia and there should be induction programmes for all new members of staff, including locums. Anaesthetists should contribute to the education and updating of midwives, operating department personnel, anaesthesia nurses and obstetricians, covering the scope and limitations of obstetric anaesthesia services.

Anaesthesia trainees

An appropriate training programme, as defined by the RCoA, should be in place for anaesthesia trainees according to their grade. A process should be in place for the formal assessment of trainees prior to allowing them to go on-call for obstetric anaesthesia with distant supervision.[16]

Anaesthetists not-in-training

Any non-consultant career-grade or staff and associate specialist anaesthetist who undertakes anaesthetic duties in the delivery suite must have been assessed by the consultant-in-charge of obstetric services as competent to perform these duties in accordance with OAA and RCoA guidelines.[10]

Provision should be made for those who cover the delivery suite on-call but do not have regular sessions there to spend time in the delivery suite in a supernumerary capacity with one of the regular obstetric anaesthetic consultants.

Midwives

Midwifery care of a labouring woman receiving epidural analgesia in labour should comply with local guidelines. The midwife must be trained to an agreed standard in regional analgesia and be aware of potential complications and their management. Midwives should be trained in high-dependency care, particularly in a tertiary referral unit with high-risk cases.

Anaesthetists should help to organise and participate in regular multi-disciplinary 'fire drills' of emergency situations, including haemorrhage and maternal collapse. All staff must be given regular access to continuing professional development opportunities.

▉ Staffing and manpower planning

Duty anaesthetist for the delivery suite

The term 'duty anaesthetist' denotes an anaesthetist who has been assessed as competent to undertake duties on the delivery suite under a specified degree of supervision (see above). The duty anaesthetist should be immediately available for the obstetric unit 24 hours a day. The duty anaesthetist should not be primarily responsible for elective obstetric work. In the busier units (that is, one or more of the following: more than 5000 deliveries/year, epidural rate higher than 35%, caesarean section rate above 25%, tertiary referral centres/high proportion of high-risk cases) it may be necessary to have two duty anaesthetists available 24 hours a day, in addition to the supervising consultant.[11]

In units that offer a 24-hour epidural service, the duty anaesthetist should be resident on site. If the anaesthetist has other responsibilities, these should be of a nature that would allow the activity to be delayed or interrupted should obstetric analgesia or anaesthesia demands arise.

Consultant anaesthetic cover

Each obstetric unit should have a named consultant anaesthetist responsible for the delivery suite 24 hours a day. That consultant should not be more than half an hour away from the delivery suite at any time. The names of all consultants covering the delivery suite should be prominently displayed and contact numbers readily available.

Each unit should have a nominated consultant-in-charge of obstetric anaesthesia services. The nominated consultant should be responsible for the organisation and audit of the service for maintaining and raising standards. As a basic minimum for any consultant-led obstetric unit, there should be ten consultant anaesthetic programmed activities or sessions a week (in addition to those for elective section lists).[10] If this degree of consultant anaesthesia cover is deemed to be excessive given the activity of the obstetric unit, this may indicate that the 'stand-alone' status of the unit is insupportable. There should be at least one consultant programmed activity available a week for antenatal referrals, whether or not a formal clinic is run.

Anaesthetic assistance

Pregnant women requiring anaesthesia have the right to the same standards of perioperative care as all other surgical patients. Skilled anaesthetic assistance is of particular importance in obstetrics. The training for all anaesthetic assistants must comply fully with current national qualification standards.[17] If such a person is not available for any reason, a registered nurse or midwife with current and effective registration, who has received equivalent anaesthesia training to a nationally or regionally recognised standard, may be employed to perform such duties. Employment of anaesthesia assistants without national accreditation is not acceptable.[13]

The anaesthesia assistant should assist the anaesthetist on a regular basis, not just occasionally, to ensure maintenance of competence. Such a person should have no other duties in the operating department at that time (thus, the midwife attending the mother and baby does not also assist the anaesthetist).

Postanaesthesia recovery staff

The training undergone by staff in recovery, whether these are midwives, nurses or operating department nurses, must be to the level recommended for general recovery facilities.[17,18] A midwife with no additional training is not adequately trained for recovery duties. Where nonmidwifery staff work in recovery as a team with midwives, it is important that basic midwifery care continues to be provided; for example, palpating the uterus and examining the lochia.

When high-dependency care is required the midwife- or nurse-to-patient ratio must be at least one midwife or nurse to two patients. Appropriately trained staff should be available 24 hours a day.

Other staff

There should be a suitably trained senior member of nursing or operating department staff with overall responsibility for the safe running of obstetric theatres. This individual should ensure all staff who work in theatre are appropriately trained and undergo regular appraisal and continuing professional development.

■ Audit

There should be an audit programme in place to audit anaesthetic complication rates, such as accidental dural puncture. There should be a system for multidisciplinary critical incident reporting in the maternity unit, which should involve the obstetric anaesthesia team. The following areas have been suggested for auditing:[19]

- adequacy of staffing
- timely anaesthesia staff involvement in the care of mothers at high risk
- information about obstetric anaesthesia and analgesia
- pain management in labour
- consent given by women during labour
- response times for provision of intrapartum analgesia and anaesthesia
- monitoring and regional analgesia

- technique of anaesthesia for caesarean section
- pain relief after caesarean section
- monitoring of obstetric patients in recovery and in the high-dependency unit
- airway and intubation problems during general anaesthesia for caesarean section
- audit programme for anaesthetic complications.

Some examples of auditable standards

Pain relief in labour
In units providing a 24-hour epidural service, the time from the anaesthetist being informed about an epidural until they are able to attend the mother should not normally exceed 30 minutes and must be within 1 hour other than in exceptional circumstances.

Anaesthesia for caesarean section
The decision to delivery interval for urgency grade 1 caesarean sections should be less than 30 minutes. Delays in elective cases should be audited. Women should receive written information about anaesthesia for caesarean section when the procedure is booked.

Future research

Research is required to:

- establish women's views about the effectiveness of various methods of pain relief during labour and the long-term impact on the newborn and the mother
- establish women's experiences of labour and access to different methods of pain relief offered
- establish the provision of antenatal assessment for women at high risk of complications to determine their suitability for various forms of pain relief during labour
- establish patient satisfaction with the local provision of epidural analgesia in various units and to explore access issues
- set quality indicators for the provision of a safe, high-quality obstetric anaesthesia service that can be used for quality accounts.

References

1. Audit Commission. *Anaesthesia Under Examination*. London: Audit Commission; 1997.
2. Royal College of Obstetricians and Gynaecologists Clinical Effectiveness Support Unit. *The National Sentinel Caesarean Section Audit Report*. London; RCOG Press; 2001.
3. National Collaborating Centre for Women's and Children's Health. *Caesarean Section*. Clinical Guideline. London: RCOG Press; 2004 [http://guidance.nice.org.uk/CG13].
4. Confidential Enquiry into Stillbirths and Deaths in Infancy. Seventh Annual Report Focusing on: Breech Presentation at Onset of Labour, Obstetric Anaesthesia: Delays and Complications, Cardiotocograph Education Survey and Sudden Unexpected Deaths in Infancy: Pathology. London: Maternal and Child Health Research Consortium; 2000 [http://www.cmace.org.uk/getattachment/%20b858e5e8-862a-4121-9348-b9284d02db1b/7th-Annual-Report.aspx].
5. Lewis G, editor. *Saving Mothers' Lives: Reviewing Maternal Deaths to Make Motherhood Safer 2003–2005. The Seventh Report of the Confidential Enquiries into Maternal Deaths in the United Kingdom*. London: CEMACH; 2007 [http://www.cmace.org.uk/getdoc/319fb647-d2c6-4b47-b6a0-a853a2f4de1b/Maternal-1.aspx].
6. Johnson RV, Lyons GR, Wilson RC, Robinson AP. Training in obstetric general anaesthesia: a vanishing art? *Anaesthesia* 2000;55:179–83.
7. Chamberlain G, Wraight A, Steer P. *Pain and its Relief in Childbirth: The Results of a National Survey Conducted by the National Birthday Trust*. Edinburgh: Churchill Livingstone; 1993.
8. Fortescue C, Wee MY, Malhotra S, Yentis SM, Holdcroft A. Is preparation for emergency obstetric anaesthesia adequate? A maternal questionnaire survey. *Int J Obstet Anesth* 2007;16:336–40.
9. Bethune L, Harper N, Lucas DN, Robinson NP, Cox M, Lilley A, et al. Complications of obstetric regional analgesia: how much information is enough? *Int J Obstet Anesth* 2004;13:30–4.
10. Association of Anaesthetists of Great Britain and Ireland; Obstetric Anaesthetists Association. OAA/AAGBI Guidelines for Obstetric Anaesthesia Services. Revised edition. London AAGBI;2005 [http://www.aagbi.org/publications/guidelines.htm#o].
11. Royal College of Anaesthetists. *Guidelines for the Provision of Anaesthetic Services*. London: RCoA; 2009 [http://www.rcoa.ac.uk/index.asp?PageID=477].
12. Royal College of Obstetricians and Gynaecologists, Royal College of Anaesthetists, Royal College of Midwives and Royal College of Paediatrics and Child Health. *Safer Childbirth: Minimum Standards for the Organisation and Delivery of Care in Labour*. London; RCOG Press; 2007 [http://www.rcog.org.uk/womens-health/clinical-guidance/safer-childbirth-minimum-standards-organisation-and-delivery-care-la].
13. Royal College of Anaesthetists, Royal College of Midwives, Royal College of Obstetricians and Gynaecologists, Royal College of Paediatrics and Child Health. *Standards for Maternity Care. Report of a Working Party*. London: RCOG Press; 2008 [http://www.rcog.org.uk/womens-health/clinical-guidance/standards-maternity-care].

14. Lewis G, Drife J, editors. *Why Mothers Die 1997–1999. The Sixth Report of the Confidential Enquiries into Maternal Deaths in the United Kingdom.* London: RCOG Press; 2002 [http://www.cmace.org.uk/Publications/CEMACH-Publications/CEMD-Publications.aspx].

15. Association of Anaesthetists of Great Britain and Ireland. *Recommendations for Standards of Monitoring During Anaesthesia and Recovery.* 4th ed. London: AAGBI; 2007 [http://www.aagbi.org/publications/guidelines.htm#s].

16. Royal College of Anaesthetists. The CCT in Anaesthesia II: Competecny Based. Basic Level (Specialty Training (ST) Years 1 and 2) Training and Assessment. A Manual for Trainees and Trainers. London: RCoA; 2007 [http://www.rcoa.ac.uk/index.asp?PageID=57].

17. Association of Anaesthetists of Great Britain and Ireland. *The Anaesthesia Team.* 3rd ed. London: AAGBI; 2010 [http://www.aagbi.org/publications/guidelines.htm#A].

18. Association of Anaesthetists of Great Britain and Ireland. *Immediate Post-anaesthetic Recovery.* London: AAGBI; 2002 [http://www.aagbi.org/publications/guidelines.htm#i].

19. Royal College of Anaesthetists. *Raising the Standard: A Compendium of Audit Recipes.* 2nd ed. London: RCoA; 2006 [http://www.rcoa.ac.uk/index.asp?PageID=125].

CHAPTER 18

Postnatal care

Rachel Liebling and Timothy Overton

Key points

✓ The partnership between healthcare professionals and the woman built in the antenatal period requires further input in the postnatal period to empower the woman, such that she can go on to guard her own health and that of her new baby both physically and emotionally, in the short and long term.

✓ Coordination of services in the postnatal period is made more difficult by the transfer of care between health professionals and clinical settings. This requires a robust local strategy that outlines the specific roles, places and timings of postnatal care provision. The central tenet is clear, written communication to ensure that women pass smoothly through this important transition into parenthood.

Introduction

Postnatal care is about the provision of a supportive environment for the woman, her baby and her family, in which they can begin their new life together. While most women and their families make this transition in an uncomplicated fashion, problems do occur and postnatal care is also about their timely recognition allowing appropriate evaluation and inter - vention. The purpose of this chapter is to provide guidance for clinicians, midwives, managers and commissioners as to the main aims and principles of postnatal care and how these should be delivered.

What women want

There has been little research into whether current models of postnatal care meet the physical and emotional needs of a new mother and her family. The needs of partners, women from diverse ethnic groups or those with physical disabilities have not been evaluated.[1] The few studies that have been performed indicate that women's perceived needs are not being met by attending healthcare professionals, with duplication of visits, conflicting advice and particular dissatisfaction with postnatal care provided by hospitals.[2,3] A survey conducted by the National Childbirth Trust showed that 10% of respondents received little or no information and 25% reported they received no emotional support.[4]

Women and their families should be treated with kindness, respect and dignity at all times. In the hospital setting, care needs to be delivered in a clean and welcoming environment with consideration for privacy when required. The views and beliefs of the woman and her family should be respected at all times and she should be intimately involved with the planning of her postnatal care. Flexibility on behalf of the healthcare professional should be encouraged allowing tailoring of postnatal care to meet the social, clinical and emotional needs of the woman and her family. All actions and interventions need to be fully discussed with the woman and the appropriate consent obtained. Good communication is essential and should be supported with evidence-based information allowing individualisation of postnatal care.

Particular attention needs to be given to providing appropriate care to women from ethnic minority groups and those with special needs, ensuring that care and information are in an accessible form. Unless specified by the woman, her partner and family should be involved in decision making, providing them with the appropriate information to support their needs.

■ National guidance and clinical guidelines

Several national guidelines on postnatal care have been referred to in the preparation of this chapter.[5–8] Guidelines for postnatal care can be considered under the following headings:

- planning the content and delivery of care
- maternal health
- infant feeding
- maintaining infant health.

Planning the content and delivery of care

Postnatal services need to be planned locally to achieve the most efficient and effective service for women and their babies. A documented, individual postnatal care plan should be identified for each woman, ideally in the antenatal period or shortly after birth. A coordinating healthcare professional needs to be identified for each woman and, because of the changing needs of the woman and her baby, this professional is likely to change over time. There should be protocols about written communication, in particular about the transfer of care between different clinical settings and from one healthcare professional to another. Information needs to be given to the woman in time for her to promote her own and her baby's health and to recognise and respond to problems. Healthcare professionals should use hand-held maternity records, postnatal care plans and child health records promoting good communication. All healthcare workers caring for mothers and babies should work within the relevant competencies developed by Skills for Health (www.skillsforhealth.org.uk).

Maternal health

Information giving

At the first postnatal contact, women should be made aware of the symptoms and signs of potentially life-threatening conditions (postpartum haemorrhage, infection, pre-eclampsia and eclampsia and thromboembolism) and a way of contacting a healthcare professional should these symptoms or signs occur. Relevant documentation should be given to the woman, including the Department of Health book *Birth to Five*[9] and the personal child health record. Information and reassurance should be offered on the physiological process of recovery after birth, normal patterns of emotional changes in the postnatal period and common health concerns as appropriate.

Mental health and wellbeing

At each postnatal contact, women should be asked about their emotional wellbeing. Together with their partners and families, they should be encouraged to inform their healthcare professional about changes in mood and emotional state. Healthcare professionals should be aware of signs and symptoms of maternal mental health. Women should be assessed for postnatal depression if symptoms of 'baby blues' have not resolved by 14 days after birth. Guidance should be given to women facilitating good mental health, including taking gentle exercise, time to rest, getting help with looking after their baby and talking to someone about their feelings.

Physical health and wellbeing

At each postnatal contact, specific enquiries should be made about the common problems encountered in the postnatal period, including perineal care, dyspareunia, headaches, fatigue, backache, constipation, haemorrhoids, faecal incontinence, urinary retention, urinary incontinence, contraception and immunisation. Anti-D should be administered within 72 hours of delivering a baby who is RhD-positive if the woman is RhD-negative and the offer of measles, mumps and rubella vaccination should be made if the mother was seronegative for rubella on antenatal screening.

Particular attention should be paid to contraception. Methods and timing of resumption of contraception should be discussed within the first week of birth. The attending healthcare professional should provide proactive assistance to women who may have difficulty accessing contraceptive care, including the provision of contact details for expert contraceptive advice if needed.

Safety

Healthcare professionals should be aware of the risks, signs and symptoms of domestic abuse and know who to contact for advice and management.

6–8-week check

At the end of the postnatal period, the healthcare professional should review the woman's physical, emotional and social wellbeing.

Infant feeding

It is important that a supportive environment for breastfeeding is encouraged. Skilled breastfeeding support should be made available regardless of the location of care through a structured programme using the Baby Friendly Initiative (www.babyfriendly.org.uk). Where postnatal care is provided in hospital, attention should be paid to facilitating an environment conducive to breastfeeding. To maximise the chance of successful breastfeeding, women should be given information on the benefits of breastfeeding within the first 24 hours after birth. Initiation of breastfeeding should be started soon after birth, ideally within the first hour following skin-to-skin contact as soon as possible after birth. Separation of the woman and her baby during this period for routine procedures should be avoided unless necessary for the immediate care of the baby. It should be recognised that additional support may be required for those women recovering from anaesthesia or caesarean section and where initial contact has been delayed.

Women who are breastfeeding should be shown how to hand-express their colostrum and store and freeze it. Breast pumps should be available in hospital, particularly for those women separated from their babies. Continuing support is essential. At each postnatal contact, the woman's experience of breastfeeding should be discussed to assess whether she is on course to breastfeed effectively, identifying the need for additional help. She will need to be educated to watch out for signs of engorgement and mastitis.

If the mother decides on formula feeding, advice should be available to ensure that it is undertaken safely to enhance infant development and health and fulfil nutritional needs.

Maintaining infant health

At each postnatal contact, parents should be offered information enabling them to assess their baby's general condition, to identify signs and symptoms of common health problems and to contact a healthcare professional or emergency service if required. An assessment of emotional attachment and parenting skills should also be made. Parents should be offered information on their baby's social capabilities, which can help parent–baby bonding, and be made aware of postnatal peer, statutory and voluntary groups and organisations in their local community.

All home visits should be used as an opportunity to assess relevant safety issues for all family members in the home environment and promote safety education. Healthcare professionals should be alert to the risk factors and signs of child abuse and if there is concern, local child protection policies should be followed. Parents should be encouraged to be present at physical examinations of their babies enabling them to learn more about their baby's needs. A complete physical examination should take place within 72 hours by a trained healthcare professional and should be repeated at 6–8 weeks of life. The newborn blood spot test should be offered to parents when their baby is 5–8 days old, a hearing screen should be completed before discharge from hospital or by week 5 and parents should be offered routine immunisations for their baby according to the schedule recommended by the Department of Health.

■ Service modelling and care pathways

Organisation and documentation

Coordinating services in the postnatal period is made more difficult by the transfer of care between health professionals and clinical settings. It is therefore important that comprehensive guidelines and protocols are established to ensure a seamless service. The organisation of 'postnatal care' may be facilitated by a multidisciplinary group, such as a postnatal working party. This may include: hospital and community midwives, obstetricians, neonatologists, general practitioners, health visitors, support workers and lay representatives. The role of this group would be as a central 'hub' to ratify local guidelines and protocols, to organise audit, to review clinical incident reports and highlighted risks, to consider and organise training requirements and competency assessment and to ensure an appropriately maintained postnatal environment.

Health professionals and roles

The role of each health professional involved should be clearly defined within the local 'postnatal care planning' document or similar. The document also needs to outline specific modes of handover from one professional to another. The individual care pathway should include the healthcare professional responsible for each stage of the postnatal 'journey' with contact details where necessary. Systems need to be in place to ensure that important information about the woman and her baby is transferred in a reliable, timely and secure manner.

Communication

The postnatal period has the potential to place a high demand on our ability to communicate. It is a period of transition, from one health professional to another, through various clinical domains and into parenthood. There is a need to consider cultural differences, language issues and vulnerable groups. While it has the potential to expose deficiencies, there is also the potential to make significant improvements and thereby a significant difference. Communication and information need to be provided in an accessible format in an approach that supports women and their families to be involved in decisions surrounding their care.

Training and education

It is essential that staff involved have the necessary training and are competency tested in certain issues pertaining to the postnatal period. The following is not an exhaustive list but should be considered: see Skills for Health (www.skillsforhealth.org.uk):

- recognising the unwell patient
- mental health
- newborn baby checks
- supporting breastfeeding
- recognising the risks, signs and symptoms of domestic and child abuse.

Environment

The postnatal environment should promote a healthy parent–infant relationship and should support the wider family. Particular attention should be made to:

- privacy, adequate rest and ready access to food and drink
- fostering a supportive approach to breastfeeding.

Audit and user feedback

The following audit criteria are taken from the National Institute for Health and Clinical Excellence clinical guideline on postnatal care.[6] *Standards for Maternity Care* also outlines specific audit standards relating to postnatal care (see standards 13–15, 18 and 19).[8]

- The existence of an individual plan that documents:
  - relevant details of history
  - healthcare professionals and their role in care
  - feeding plans
  - advice and management at each contact
  - emotional wellbeing.

- Local protocols detailing communication during the transfer of care:
  - method of communication
  - relevant items of information
  - method of handover of care plan.

- Information given at first postnatal contact of the signs and symptoms of potentially life-threatening conditions to mother and baby and who to contact:
  - evidence in the care plan
  - case note audit of cases of late, life-threatening re-admissions of mother or infant.

- All maternity care providers should implement and evaluate externally a structured programme that encourages breastfeeding using the Baby Friendly Initiative as a minimum standard. There should be evidence of implementation of the scheme including:
  - training of staff
  - implementation of Baby Friendly Initiative principles
  - external audit.

- User feedback may be particularly helpful regarding the users' overall perspective of their 'postnatal stay' with attention paid to:
  - approach by staff members
  - food and hygiene
  - information.

Special issues related to service delivery

Various neonatal screening tests are carried out in the postnatal period:

- newborn hearing tests
- blood spot tests for phenylketonuria, congenital hypothyroidism, cystic fibrosis, MCADD (medium-chain acyl dehydrogenase deficiency) and sickle cell disease
- newborn physical examination for developmental dislocation of the hip, congenital heart disease, cryptorchidism, congenital cataracts and other structural eye anomalies and congenital malformations.

Appropriate training and coordination with allied services is required to ensure a standardised approach and service.

Future research

- What women want in the postnatal period: minimal evaluation has been carried out as to whether current models of postnatal care meet the needs of women and babies in today's times.
- Routine monitoring of the weight of babies: does routine monitoring of the weight of all low-risk babies during the first 6–8 weeks after birth reduce the incidence of serious morbidities?
- Evaluation of the Baby Friendly Initiative: what is the impact of the use of the Baby Friendly Initiative on breastfeeding uptake and duration?
- The effect of peer support on severity of postnatal depression: is the severity of postnatal depression among women who are socially isolated reduced by the provision of peer social support compared with standard care?

References

1. MacArthur C, Winter HR, Bick DE, Knowles H, Lilford R, Henderson C, et al. Effects of redesigned community postnatal care on women's health 4 months after birth: a cluster randomised controlled trial. *Lancet* 2002;359:378–85.
2. Audit Commission for Local Authorities and the National Health Service in England and Wales. *First Class Delivery: Improving Maternity Services in England and Wales*. Abingdon: Audit Commission Publications; 1997.
3. Murphy-Black T. Postnatal Care at Home: A Descriptive Study of Mothers' Needs and the Maternity Services. Edinburgh: Nursing Research Unit, University of Edinburgh; 1989.
4. National Childbirth Trust. *Reconfiguring Maternity Services: Views of User Representatives*. London: National Childbirth Trust; 2003.
5. Demott K, Bick D, Norman R, Ritchie G, Turnbull N, Adams C, et al. *Clinical Guidelines and Evidence Review For Post Natal Care: Routine Post Natal Care Of Recently Delivered Women And Their Babies*. London: National Collaborating Centre for Primary Care and Royal College Of General Practitioners; 2006 [http://www.nice.org.uk/guidance/CG37].
6. National Institute for Health and Clinical Excellence. *Routine Postnatal Care of Women and Their Babies*. Clinical Guideline CG37. London: NICE; 2006 [http://www.nice.org.uk/guidance/CG37].
7. National Institute for Health and Clinical Excellence. *Routine Postnatal Care of Women and Their Babies*. Quick Reference Guide. London: NICE; 2006 [http://www.nice.org.uk/guidance/CG37].

8. Royal College of Anaesthetists, Royal College of Midwives, Royal College of Obstetricians and Gynaecologists, Royal College of Paediatrics and Child Health. *Standards for Maternity Care. Report of a Working Party*. London: RCOG Press; 2008 [http://www.rcog.org.uk/womens-health/clinical-guidance/standards-maternity-care].
9. Department of Health. Birth to Five. London: DH; 2009 [http://www.dh.gov.uk/en/Publicationsandstatistics/Publications/PublicationsPolicyAndGuidance/DH_107303].

CHAPTER 19

Supporting families who experience adverse outcomes during pregnancy

Judith Schott, Alix Henley and Gordon Smith

Key points

✓ Pregnancy loss, stillbirth and early neonatal death are major bereavements that have lasting effects on parents and their families.

✓ Gestation is not an accurate predictor of the length or depth of the parents' grief.

✓ Good care cannot alleviate parents' pain but poor or insensitive care makes things worse.

✓ Parents value privacy, including for discussions, empathy, good clear communication and sensitive support to help them to make their own informed choices.

✓ There should be dedicated facilities for parents whose baby dies.

✓ All that parents take home with them are their memories. The staff who cared for them form a large part of those memories. Parents appreciate staff who demonstrate respect and care for their baby as an individual, who show that they care and who offer opportunities to create memories of their baby.

✓ Bereaved parents need special care and attention during and after all subsequent pregnancies and births.

✓ Staff need multidisciplinary training on supporting and communicating with bereaved parents to ensure that care is consistent and seamless. All staff who care for bereaved parents also need access to a range of support systems.

✓ There should be clear pathways between secondary and primary care teams to help ensure continuing care and support.

▇ Introduction

The death of a baby during pregnancy or birth is a major bereavement and has long-lasting effects. The trauma of the loss can damage physical and mental health, relationships, careers and incomes.[1] The quality of care that parents receive at these times has a profound effect on their wellbeing and that of their families, both now and in the future. Good care cannot remove the pain of their grief, but poor care makes everything worse. This chapter is based mainly on *Pregnancy Loss and the Death of a Baby: Guidelines for Professionals*.[2] The Sands guidelines are based on a combination of research, best practice and the views and experiences of bereaved parents.

▇ What women want

It is essential that staff make no comparisons or assumptions about the significance to the parents of their loss. A shorter gestation is not necessarily less damaging: there were no significant differences in grief responses between women who had a miscarriage, a stillbirth or a neonatal death.[3-5]

Understanding and empathy

Women want to be cared for by skilled staff who show empathy and support for them and their partner and who give them privacy and time. They appreciate staff who know how grief can affect people's ability to listen, absorb information and make decisions. They want staff to ask about, respect and accept their feelings and to be sensitive to any religious and cultural requirements. It is important that staff treat their baby's body with respect and tenderness and use the baby's name if one was given. They also want staff to be aware of the possible impact of the loss on other children and on grandparents.

Excellent communication

Communication is the bedrock of good care. All communication with parents should be clear, broken down into manageable chunks and in nontechnical language. Staff should avoid euphemisms because these may confuse parents. Parents want:

- privacy for all discussions with staff
- time to take in information, to clarify, ask questions and have information repeated when necessary
- a trained interpreter whenever required
- clear written information about what they need to do and their options. This should be in the main languages spoken locally and take cultural and religious beliefs and sensitivities into account.

Prompt and effective communication between staff is essential. This saves parents having to tell staff what has happened and avoids unintended but hurtful assumptions and remarks. Sands 'teardrop' stickers on the front of notes are an effective way of alerting staff.

There must also be prompt communication between:

- different departments and units; for instance, if a mother travels to a fetal medicine unit for investigations or feticide
- the staff who seek consent for a postmortem and the pathologist who will perform it; wherever possible, this should be a perinatal pathologist[6]
- the hospital and the woman's general practitioner and primary care team; for example, the latter should be informed of the death of a baby within one working day.[6]

The mother's lead midwife is normally responsible for communication with other team members and with the mother.[6]

National guidance and clinical guidelines

Several publications are available that provide guidance and set standards for the care of women and families experiencing pregnancy loss.[2,6–11]

Service modelling and care pathways

Women and their partners should have as much choice about their care as possible. The death of a baby often removes parents' feelings of autonomy and certainty. It is important to enable them to retain as much control as possible over what happens to them and to their baby. However, most parents have little idea of the decisions and choices that they can make. They should be offered explanations of all their options and given opportunities to make informed choices. They should also be given as much time as possible to decide what would be best for them: there are no right or wrong decisions, just decisions that parents can live with.[12] Staff should make it clear to parents that they have the right to change their minds, provided that events and timing allow.

Clear pathways between secondary care and the primary care team are essential to ensure that bereaved parents receive good care at all times.[6]

Early pregnancy units with dedicated ultrasound facilities should be accessible to women experiencing an early miscarriage. Women who have had three miscarriages should be offered referral for specialist care.[6,7]

When an abnormality is seen on ultrasound or a woman presents with a threatened miscarriage or reduced fetal movements, she should receive prompt assessment and prompt results.[13]

Women having an early miscarriage should be given a choice about management options.[7,14] Ideally, women having a late miscarriage should be able to choose between the gynaecology ward and the labour ward. If they are not cared for on the labour ward, they must be cared for by skilled staff who are trained to:

- deliver and handle the baby sensitively
- offer practical and emotional support during and after labour
- offer the same choices about creating memories as the mother would receive on the labour ward.[6]

After a late miscarriage, stillbirth or early neonatal death, parents should be offered opportunities to:

- see and hold their baby and collect mementoes such as photos and hand- and footprints
- take their baby's body home for a short time
- discuss whether they want a postmortem examination; the nature and outcome of discussions about consent to a postmortem should be recorded
- choose and possibly participate in a funeral organised by the hospital or organise the funeral themselves.

Parents should be offered privacy in waiting rooms, ultrasound and other departments, clinics and wards, away from women with straightforward pregnancies and healthy babies. While they are in hospital, each mother should be offered a separate room with en suite facilities and space for her partner to stay.[6]

Before she leaves hospital, the mother should be given an appointment for a postnatal visit, as well as a separate appointment to receive and discuss postmortem results. The RCOG standard states that the placental and postmortem histology results should be available within 6 weeks of the examination.[6] For parents, it is important that their discussion with the lead obstetrician or paediatrician about these results takes place as soon as is practicably possible.

Many parents hope that the postmortem will explain why their baby died and some will want to know the possible implications for future pregnancies. Some parents may welcome an opportunity to discuss whether and when to try for another baby. Others may not be ready to think about this. If appropriate, parents should be offered referral for genetic counselling.

Parents who have had a childbearing loss need special care and consideration during and after all subsequent pregnancies and births. Often, no amount of reassurance can remove their fear that the same thing might happen again. They should be offered extra care, attention and monitoring. Some women may prefer to attend a different unit or be cared for by a different group of staff. Others welcome care from familiar and trusted staff.

▮ Special issues related to service delivery

Each woman's loss is unique but parents in certain situations face additional trauma and, often, painful decisions.

Serious or lethal fetal anomalies

When a serious fetal abnormality is diagnosed, the mother has to decide what to do. The decision as to whether to terminate is always difficult, especially if it involves feticide, which may require travelling to another unit. Parents whose baby has a lethal abnormality may refuse feticide, hoping that they may be able to see and hold their baby for a short time before he or she dies.

The prospect of induction and labour that will culminate in a stillbirth is daunting. Even when women feel that termination is the right decision for them, they may experience grief that is as intense as that of women who have had a spontaneous perinatal loss.[4] They need sensitive support and understanding and should be offered all the choices that are open to parents who have a spontaneous loss.

Most women who choose to continue the pregnancy knowing that their baby will be severely ill or disabled or will die at birth find it distressing to share waiting rooms or attend antenatal classes with women who have straightforward pregnancies. They should be offered antenatal care away from the normal clinic with staff who know them and who provide support, care and antenatal education tailored to their specific needs. They should be cared for by familiar staff during labour and have a single room while the mother is in hospital. If the baby is likely to be admitted to the neonatal unit, the parents should be able to visit and meet the staff before the birth.

Babies born at the borderline of viability

Babies born at the borderline of viability present clinicians and parents with difficult dilemmas. If there is time before the birth, parents should have an opportunity to talk to a senior paediatrician about the realistic prospects for their baby, what to expect when she or he is born and, depending on the gestation and the condition, what care might be offered. If it is decided not to institute active treatment, the parents should be assured that their baby will receive 'comfort' or palliative care for as long as she or he is alive. A care plan for the baby should be drawn up, agreed with the parents and filed in the mother's notes. However, the baby's condition cannot be properly assessed until after the birth, so staff should tell the parents that the care plan may be adapted when the paediatrician has examined the baby and decides what care would be in her or his best interests.[15] Parents find it easier to trust the views of doctors who are sensitive and open and who explain simply and honestly what would be in their baby's best interests. If agreement cannot be reached, a second opinion should be offered. If there is no time for detailed discussion before the birth, the parents should be informed as soon as possible what to expect when their baby is born and what sort of care is planned for him or her. If no care plan has been agreed and no senior paediatrician is available when a very premature baby is born showing signs of life, the nurse or midwife 'must use their professional judgment as to whether the baby is capable of survival' and if so 'should instigate resuscitative measures' until the baby is assessed by senior medical staff.

Multiple pregnancy

Parents who have more than one baby may face conflicting emotions and divided loyalties if one or more survive and one or more die. They are likely to be struggling with grief and, at the same time, with hope tinged with anxiety for the surviving baby. It is important that staff remember that the survival of one or more babies does not 'compensate' parents for the baby or babies who die.

In the case of a multiple birth in which, for example, one baby is healthy and the other cannot live, parents often feel torn. They may appreciate reassurance that there will be plenty of time afterwards to make up for what they may feel is neglect of the healthier baby, and encouragement to make the most of this time with the baby who is unlikely to survive. They may want to create memories (which might include a photo of all the babies together) so that they, and in the future the surviving child, have some tangible evidence of the baby who died.

■ Training

Most training for staff who care for bereaved parents should be multi-disciplinary. Training on grief should include:

- awareness that the experience of grief is much more chaotic and tumultuous than theories of grief imply
- possible differences between the experience and the expression of grief[16]
- potential personal, cultural or religious preferences.[6]

Training on communication skills should include:

- listening skills, including taking seriously what women and their partners say
- breaking bad news
- giving clear, succinct information using everyday language and avoiding euphemisms
- communicating across language barriers and using an interpreter
- enabling informed choice and supporting parents in making decisions
- requesting consent for postmortem examination (this should always be done by a consultant or in the presence of a consultant)

- familiarity with all the relevant hospital policies and procedures, including provision for funerals and memorial services, and sensitive disposal of fetal tissue.

Staffing and manpower planning

Staffing levels should ensure that parents receive continuity of carers. Carers must have training to enable them to support grieving parents, and must themselves be well supported. Junior and inexperienced staff must be supervised, especially during busy periods and at night.

Specialist bereavement staff should train and supervise junior and inexperienced staff. They should also have input into all protocols, policies and procedures that are relevant to the care of bereaved parents. If the unit offers funerals, specialist bereavement staff should be involved in agreeing the content of contracts with local funeral directors, crematoria and burial grounds, and in monitoring the provision of contracted services. There should be increased provision of perinatal pathologists.[9]

Providing good care to bereaved parents is extremely demanding. A range of support systems should be in place. The organisational culture should recognise that it is both responsible and professional for staff to seek support when they need it.

Audit

The bereavement service as a whole should be audited regularly to ensure that it provides comprehensive, culturally sensitive management and support for families who have experienced an early or mid-pregnancy loss, stillbirth or neonatal death.[2] There should also be an audit of provision, which should identify:

- the proportion of women seen by dedicated bereavement coordinators, usually specialist midwives, who offer support following late miscarriage, stillbirth or neonatal death
- the proportion of women experiencing early pregnancy loss managed in a dedicated early pregnancy unit with dedicated ultrasound facilities and suitable expertise
- the support of and provision for parents who choose to continue their pregnancy following the diagnosis of a serious or lethal abnormality
- the availability of dedicated separate facilities for grieving families at the time of and after a loss

- specialist transport services for transferring babies' bodies for postmortem examination from units lacking onsite perinatal pathology and the length of time that elapses before the body is returned
- the proportion of staff who care for parents who experience pregnancy or childbearing loss who have received appropriate training
- the provision of trained interpreters at key points of care
- the percentage of women with three or more miscarriages, and the number who are offered a referral to a specialist recurrent miscarriage clinic
- the percentage of general practitioners and community midwives who are informed within one working day of a late miscarriage, stillbirth or neonatal death
- the length of time taken to deliver postmortem results to the lead clinician
- the percentage of parents offered an appointment to discuss postmortem results within 6 weeks of their baby's death.

In addition, each neonatal death and stillbirth should be 'subject to audit' and thoroughly investigated, not to apportion blame but to identify contributory factors and indicators of risk that may have been missed during the mother's antenatal or intrapartum care.

Feedback on care should be sought regularly from bereaved parents and support groups such as Antenatal Results and Choices,[12] the Miscarriage Association and Sands. Maternity Services Liaison Committees are also well placed to gather the views and comments of parents who represent those whose babies have died.

References

1. Sands: Stillbirth and Neonatal Death Charity. *Saving Babies' Lives Report 2009*. London: Sands; 2009 [http://www.why17.org/fileadmin/content/About_Sands/03520_Saving_babies_lives_watermarked.pdf].
2. Schott J, Henley A, Kohner N. *Pregnancy Loss and the Death of a Baby: Guidelines for Professionals*. London: Sands; 2007.
3. Mander R. *Loss and Bereavement in Childbearing*. 2nd ed. London: Routledge; 2005.
4. Zeanah C, Dailey J, Rosenblatt M, Saller DN Jr. Do women grieve after terminating pregnancies because of fetal anomalies? A controlled investigation. *Obstet Gynecol* 1993;82:270–5.

5. Peppers L, Knapp R. Maternal reactions to involuntary fetal/infant death. *Psychiatry* 1980;43:155–9.
6. Royal College of Anaesthetists, Royal College of Midwives, Royal College of Obstetricians and Gynaecologists, Royal College of Paediatrics and Child Health. *Standards for Maternity Care. Report of a Working Party*. London: RCOG Press; 2008 [http://www.rcog.org.uk/womens-health/clinical-guidance/standards-maternity-care].
7. Royal College of Obstetricians and Gynaecologists. *Standards for Gynaecology. Report of a Working Party*. London: RCOG; 2008 [http://www.rcog.org.uk/womens-health/clinical-guidance/standards-gynaecology].
8. Royal College of Obstetricians and Gynaecologists. *The Management of Early Pregnancy Loss*. Green-top Guideline No 25. London: RCOG; 2006 [http://www.rcog.org.uk/womens-health/clinical-guidance/management-early-pregnancy-loss-green-top-25].
9. Royal College of Obstetricians and Gynaecologists; Royal College of Pathologists. *Fetal and Perinatal Pathology: Report of a Joint Working Party*. London: RCOG; 2001 [http://www.rcog.org.uk/womens-health/clinical-guidance/fetal-and-perinatal-pathology].
10. Royal College of Obstetricians and Gynaecologists. *Disposal Following Pregnancy Loss Before 24 Weeks of Gestation*. Good Practice No. 5. London: RCOG; 2005 [http://www.rcog.org.uk/womens-health/clinical-guidance/disposal-following-pregnancy-loss-24-weeks-gestation].
11. Royal College of Obstetricians and Gynaecologists. *Recurrent Miscarriage, Investigation and Treatment of Couples*. Green-top Guideline No. 17. London: RCOG; 2003 [http://www.rcog.org.uk/womens-health/clinical-guidance/investigation-and-treatment-couples-recurrent-miscarriage-green-top-].
12. Antenatal Results and Choices. *Supporting Parents' Decisions: A Handbook for Professionals*. London: ARC; 2005.
13. National Institute for Health and Clinical Excellence. *Antenatal Care: Routine Care for the Healthy Pregnant Woman*. NICE Clinical Guideline 62. London: NICE; 2008 [http://guidance.nice.org.uk/CG62].
14. Smith LF, Frost J, Levitas R, Bradley H, Garcia J. Women's experiences of three early miscarriage management options: A qualitative study. *Br J Gen Pract* 2006:56:198–205.
15. British Association of Perinatal Medicine. Fetuses and Newborn Infants at the Threshold of Viability: A Framework for Practice Memorandum. London: BAPM; 2000.
16. Cowles KV. Cultural perspectives on grief: an expanded concept analysis. *J Adv Nurs* 1996;23:287–94.

CHAPTER 20
The maternity dashboard

Edward Morris

Key points

✓ The maternity dashboard is primarily a tool to record maternity data in an 'at-a-glance' format to aid the clinical governance process.
✓ Important additional benefits of the dashboard include support of CQUIN, other audit needs, the commissioning process and the operational and strategic needs of maternity units.
✓ Use of existing data sources optimises the reliability of a dashboard and the speed and efficiency of production.
✓ Several different types of dashboard exist, from manually completed systems to spreadsheet macro-based and to automatic interactive web-based systems.

▓ Introduction

One of the cornerstones of modern clinical governance is using data to inform risk management processes. Most units have electronic maternity data systems that have been evolving over the past 15–20 years and are able to provide data to facilitate risk management decisions. More recent versions of these maternity software packages provide impressive ways of manipulating data to be displayed in numerical and graphic forms.

The main drawback of such systems is that they are resource-hungry in terms of the time required to enter the data at the time of birth. However, most units accept this use of midwifery time as a vital part of the care of women with the expectation that the system provides relevant data that are useful. Unfortunately, the process for extracting the data is not only frequently difficult and time-consuming, it also requires staff with an understanding of information technology and maternity care.

Another consideration is that maternity systems do not collect all the data that are required for each of the domains of risk management. Good examples of these deficient areas are incident reporting, complaints and staffing numbers.

This chapter explores the reasoning behind the need for an up-to-date, easy-to-use data demonstration system, the first use of a maternity dashboard in England and subsequent developments. These innovations include a simple way of using data from maternity packages and an electronic dashboard system that extracts data from maternity software and other data packages relevant to the specialty.

What women want

All recent surveys of women have indicated that they want assurance that the maternity unit where they are planning to give birth is not only safe but also adequately staffed. They would also like to have an assurance that systems are in place so that organisations are proactive in putting corrective actions in place if and when things do go wrong. The maternity dashboard captures information prospectively on such key clinical indicators as are relevant to the day-to-day outcomes in labour. Such readily available performance figures can then reasonably be used to inform women as well as to support the local governance process.

Definitions

The first mention of dashboards within the medical literature was in their ability to cause fractures in road traffic accidents; therefore, 'dashboard' is a definition that clearly needs updating. Since 1993, when one of the first publications describing how a dashboard can be used to report quality of care to the board of a healthcare organisation appeared,[1] there has been a slow rise in the number of publications demonstrating the potential for improvements in safety and quality of care that can arise from the use of a dashboard. A current definition of a clinical dashboard could therefore be 'a visual display of information and outcomes relevant to the care system being monitored which can be arranged on a single device or screen that results in user response where appropriate'.

Types of dashboard

Most clinical directors are aware of the use of 'dashboards' to demonstrate performance in terms of patient throughput and financial efficiency. What differentiates an otherwise relatively dry spreadsheet from a dashboard is the fact that there is a system for indicating 'at a glance' whether the numbers within the cell show performance that is acceptable or reaches an alert level. The most commonly used methodology for this is the use of a red, amber, green (RAG) system, where a green colour to a cell shows acceptable performance, amber raises concern and red is the action level. It is important therefore to be aware that several different types of 'dashboard' exist.

Clinical dashboards are a relatively new phenomenon. As the prime motivator for a unit to have a functioning maternity dashboard is to improve safety, it is important that it provides meaningful data that are relevant to the unit and also to commissioning bodies such as primary care trusts (PCTs) and strategic health authorities (SHAs). The use of a maternity dashboard is not yet a mandatory national requirement, but some PCTs now require a locally specified maternity dashboard to be in place to supply indicators of quality of care for the Commissioning for Quality and Innovation (CQUIN) payment framework such as the NHS Commissioning Board and the general practitioner-led local commissioning consortia. The use of a maternity dashboard is not yet a mandatory national requirement but, in due course, outcome indicator-based information generated through maternity dashboards could be used to support the CQUIN payment framework.

Potential uses of a maternity dashboard

The primary reason for the use of a dashboard should be to provide information, to support governance and to reduce risk. Other benefits that should be considered are the fact that the data collected can be used as part of the audit for processes such as the Clinical Negligence Scheme for Trusts (CNST), CQUIN and, more recently, quality, innovation, productivity and prevention (QIPP).

National guidance and clinical guidelines

At present, no national guidance exists as to how to produce a maternity dashboard. The process of dashboard development is a rapidly growing area and this chapter aims to outline the essentials for a successful end product.

Design and contents of the maternity dashboard

One of the first documented uses of a maternity dashboard in England was in the process of helping a unit in difficulty.[2] Factors that were identified as contributing to this unit's problems, as well as other indices of good clinical governance, were incorporated into the design. Each individual factor or metric that made up this dashboard was part of one of the following four domains:

- clinical activity
- workforce
- clinical outcomes
- risk incidents, complaints or patient satisfaction surveys.

It is important that any modern dashboard uses these domains as its backbone. While the subsequent metrics within the dashboard are not compulsory, the following metrics are given as illustrations of potential contents for each domain:

- clinical activity
- antenatal bookings per month
- normal birth rate
- caesarean sections (emergency and elective)
- instrumental deliveries
- number of times unit closed or women diverted
- workforce
- episodes of staff shortage leading to clinical pressures
- numbers of midwives rostered
- women delivering with one-to-one midwifery care
- consultant presence on delivery floor
- attendance at mandatory training
- clinical outcomes
- maternal morbidity, such as major haemorrhage, eclampsia, third- and fourth-degree perineal tears

- neonatal morbidity, such as brachial plexus injury, meconium aspiration and hypoxic ischaemic encephalopathy
- admissions to neonatal and/or adult intensive care
- risk incidents, complaints or patient satisfaction surveys
- numbers of complaints from specific clinical areas such as the community, clinics, delivery suite and ward areas
- incident reporting data from in-house incident reporting system.

Sources of data

A key consideration when producing a dashboard is to make the collection of data and entry into the dashboard as straightforward as possible with minimal drain on staff time. Data concerning clinical outcomes alone are likely to be already available within an electronic data recording system and their entry into the dashboard is likely to be a matter of setting up an appropriate data report to be produced each month. Other important sources of data can also be obtained from many of the pre-existing electronic systems within NHS trusts. Such systems relevant to maternity include:

- neonatal intensive care electronic care records can provide neonatal outcomes, admission rates and length of stay
- patient administration systems can provide details about transfer to other ward areas and near-live bed occupancy
- incident reporting software is increasingly becoming electronic and will provide numbers of complaints and other incident triggers predetermined by the obstetric unit
- electronic staff management software ('e-rostering') is currently in use in a small number of trusts. Data from e-rostering can provide staffing levels if these are selected for inclusion in the dashboard.

Whatever the source of data, it is important for a unit to be aware that not all data are available electronically and that some information may need to be entered manually.

The RAG system

Any unit that elects to set up a maternity dashboard needs to set the goals for the dashboard using the RAG system. The examples provided in the RCOG Good Practice document were specific to the unit being studied and it is important that units are aware that they will need to set their own RAG limits.[2]

Informing the RAG limits is best achieved by performing a retrospective analysis of the proposed outcomes that are to be monitored in the dashboard, comparing performance with regional or national indices and then setting provisional limits for the dashboard. Another way of monitoring performance is to use cumulative sum (CUSUM) analysis, which is a cumulative performance measure over time in which a probability testing procedure is sequentially applied to the data, assessing 'current performance' against a specific baseline or target performance level.[3]

What to do with the dashboard

The main output of the dashboard is to inform the governance process and so it should be reviewed frequently. Units already using a dashboard tend to review it monthly in directorate risk management or governance meetings. Many trust boards are interested in the output of the maternity dashboard and it is therefore important that the dashboard becomes part of the trust reporting structure, which will help increase awareness of maternity issues by the board.

Regular reviews of the dashboard will provide vital information to help early detection of adverse changes in outcomes and attempts can be made to extract other information from the data to identify reasons and contributing factors to these changes.

A simple example of how a dashboard may help is to observe a fall in the normal birth rate over several months. If there was a concomitant fall in women receiving one-to-one care in labour, it would be appropriate to investigate any rostering difficulties. A clinical example would be a member of staff browsing the dashboard and noticing an increase in neonatal intensive care unit admissions of term babies (Figure 20.1). This would be reported to the risk management team for further investigation of dashboard data to investigate possible reasons for the admissions. Another example would be a sustained increase in unit closures with a reduction of midwifery staff numbers rostered per shift (Figure 20.2). These data presented early to the trust board may facilitate the early approval of a business case to appoint additional midwifery staff.

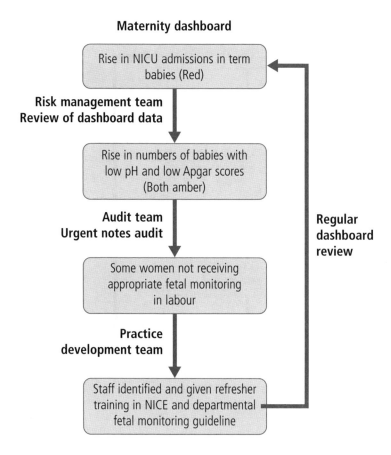

Maternity dashboard

Figure 20.1 Use of the maternity dashboard in a clinical scenario

Training

For units that already have an information technology (IT) midwife or other staff dedicated to the maintenance of the electronic maternity packages, very little additional training is required. Additional time will be required during the set-up phase of the project followed by monthly extraction of the required data fields from the software packages. The preferred approach is to limit the responsibility of dashboard production to a core team with the aim of a streamlined and efficient monthly output.

It is recognised that production of a monthly dashboard may require the collection of data currently not being captured; this is especially relevant to units that do not currently collect data electronically. In these circumstances, it is recommended that rather than producing a paper

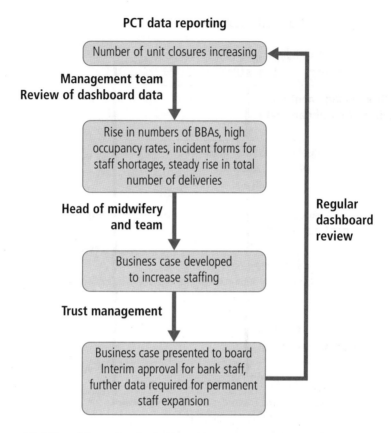

Figure 20.2 Use of the maternity dashboard in a management scenario

dashboard, the data are recorded on a centrally located electronic spreadsheet. This can be used not only to inform initial versions of the dashboard but also to provide data for some of the forthcoming developments in dashboard design (see **Future research** below).

Using a spreadsheet computer program to combine the data and performance limits is the accepted means of displaying the information. Cells of data contain numbers and are filled with one of the RAG colours to highlight whether performance is satisfactory or not. This process has traditionally been performed manually for small lists of metrics, but as discussed above this can be resource-hungry. Most trust IT departments can be briefed on the production of such a spreadsheet that is relatively straightforward to complete and can then provide training to staff in dashboard data entry and production.

Staffing and manpower planning

It is unlikely that the development of a maternity dashboard will require a significant expansion in staff. However, training of clinical staff with IT skills to provide clinical input into the set-up and subsequent running of the dashboard is vital. 'Pure' IT staff are appropriate for technical and training aspects but often require clinical steer throughout the process. 'Pure' adminstrative and clerical staff may be used to collect routine data or input the data systems. If such systems are used, the overall clinical lead for the dashboard needs to be satisfied that the quality of data entry systems is such that staff entering the data without clinical knowledge not only enter data correctly but are also unable to corrupt existing data.

Where the dashboard identifies clear links between clinical outcomes and staffing issues, the data should, as discussed previously, be used to facilitate the manpower planning process, both at directorate and trust levels.

Audit

The dashboard is a continuous process of audit and, if considered at the beginning of its design, could be made to develop into a system for collecting some of the audit requirements for CNST. Units that develop a useful and informative dashboard should monitor its use and record carefully how the unit responds to information from the dashboard.

Future research

Automated or semi-automated maternity dashboards are areas of very active development at present.

References

1. Bader BS. CQI progress reports: the dashboard approach provides a better way to keep board informed about quality. *Healthc Exec* 1993;8:8–11.
2. Royal College of Obstetricians and Gynaecologists. *Maternity Dashboard: Clinical Performance and Governance Scorecard.* Good Practice No 7. London: RCOG; 2008 [http://www.rcog.org.uk/womens-health/clinical-guidance/maternity-dashboard-clinical-performance-and-governance-score-card].
3. Sibanda T, Sibanda N, Siassakos D, Sivananthan S, Robinson Z, Winter C, et al. Prospective evaluation of a continuous monitoring and quality-improvement system for reducing adverse neonatal outcomes. *Am J Obstet Gynecol* 2009;201:480.e1–6.

CHAPTER 21

Commissioning for regional maternity services: an example from the East of England

Lyn McIntyre and Boon H Lim

Key points

✓ The design of the regional clinical service must be clinically led, with input from clinicians, users of the service and commissioners.
✓ Solutions must be evidence-based to develop high-quality care, with patients at the centre of the development.

Introduction

The National Health Service (NHS) in the UK celebrated its 60th anni - versary in 2008. It has undergone significant changes since its inception, but 2008 saw the most significant review of the NHS in England. This was led by Professor Lord Ara Darzi, a consultant surgeon who was appointed Health Minister, and resulted in the publication *NHS Next Stage Review*.[1] This was an ambitious project involving the ten strategic health authorities (SHAs) in England and placed clinicians at the forefront of leading the change. Each SHA was tasked to develop its vision for clinical services for the next decade to deliver the best possible health service for the 21st century.

In the East of England, the SHA (NHS East of England) set up ten clinical pathway groups in early 2008 to design the clinical vision for all aspects of health care from the newborn period to the end of life. The aim of the vision was to deliver 'the best health service' in England. The Maternity and Newborn Clinical Pathway Group was one of the groups tasked to develop the vision for the best possible maternity and newborn services for the Region.

The pathway group was clinically led, with an obstetrician as the chair, supported by a programme manager and a working group comprising 30 clinicians, commissioners and user representatives. The group examined all the available evidence and models of good practice to come up with their recommendations (Box 21.1).

Box 21.1 Priorities for implementation of the Maternity and Newborn Clinical Programme Board for the East of England

- Ensure that all 17 acute trusts will keep an obstetric unit, with a co-located midwife-led unit.
- Guarantee one-to-one midwifery care in established labour and recruit the necessary number of additional midwives to do this.
- Maximise care for ill babies by increasing the numbers of level three intensive-care cots and level one special care units and reducing the number of level two high-dependency units.
- Offer preconception care to women with pre-existing health problems and lifestyle issues.
- Increase the overall number of NHS-funded in vitro fertilisation cycles against standard criteria.
- Guarantee women direct access to midwives and choice of antenatal care.
- Promote normality of birth and guarantee women choice on where to give birth, based on an assessment of safety for mother and baby.
- Guarantee choice of postnatal care to women, especially those most in need.
- Establish networks covering maternity and neonatal services.

Upon conclusion of the work of all the clinical pathway groups, NHS East of England launched the vision for the development of healthcare for the next decade in the summer of 2008. This programme was called

Towards the Best, Together.[2] This is the vision for the NHS in the East of England, setting out how health and healthcare services should be improved, now and over the next decade, to meet the overall goal of being the best health service in England. It is the culmination of the work of hundreds of clinicians and NHS professionals.

This was indeed an ambitious project but it was considered to be the best opportunity to modernise the NHS to make it fit for purpose for the future.

■ Translating the vision into action

The purpose of the clinical pathway group was to develop the strategy and vision that was clinically led and evidence-based. The work, having been completed, was then handed over to the clinical programme board to take forward the implementation of the recommendations. Ten clinical programme boards were established in December 2008 to take forward the pledges in the vision, with responsibility for driving forward change, encouraging innovation and monitoring progress.

The vision set out by the Maternity and Newborn Clinical Programme Board in the *Towards the Best, Together* report is to plan and deliver a maternity and newborn service for the East of England that will ensure the best outcome for mothers and babies. The key aim is to improve the quality of service, safety, outcomes and satisfaction for all women through offering informed choice around the types of care throughout pregnancy, birth and postnatally.

The clinical pathway group is led by a clinical chair who is an obstetrician and a programme lead who provides professional and administrative support. The membership of the clinical programme board includes a range of key stakeholders including clinicians from maternity, neonatal services and general practice, commissioners, users, NHS East of England and Public Health. It is supported by a chief executive from a primary care trust and an executive director of the SHA who is the chief nurse. This ensures that not only is the group clinically led but there is good engagement between the commissioners who purchase the service and the SHA that develops the strategy and monitors the provision of clinical services in the region.

The vision outlined is underpinned by national policy documents, including *Maternity Matters*.[3] This builds on the maternity services commitment outlined in *Our Health, Our Care, Our Say*[4] and is an important step towards meeting Maternity Standard 11 set out in the National Service Framework for Children, Young People and Maternity Services.[5]

One of the main priorities is to implement recommendations that guarantee that women will be provided with a choice of how to access antenatal care, a choice of place of birth and a choice of place of postnatal care.

Key areas of work and achievements

It is natural for staff to feel threatened whenever there is any review of services. By being able to guarantee that all the 17 acute (provider) trusts in the region will continue to have a maternity unit provided the assurance needed and allowed staff to focus on healthcare delivery without any distraction.

Fertility services

The clinical programme board worked closely with the specialised commissioning group for fertility services to ensure that the 'postcode lottery' for access to in vitro fertilisation (IVF) services is removed. The provision of IVF treatment for eligible couples is now compliant with the National Institute for Health and Clinical Excellence (NICE) guideline and is uniform across the East of England Region.[6] All eligible couples are now able to access NHS-funded IVF treatment for three cycles of treatment.

The current focus of the work of the clinical programme board is on prepregnancy care, maternal mental health, workforce, clinical pathways, normality of birth and the development of a maternity dashboard.

Prepregnancy care

The most important way to achieve good outcomes in pregnancy is to ensure that the woman is in the best possible health before she embarks on her pregnancy.[7] This is clearly a challenging agenda, as it involves all aspects of social and health advice. Nevertheless, the clinical programme board identified this as an important area to address and is working closely with the clinical programme boards for long-term conditions and mental health and the Staying Healthy group to promote healthy lifestyle advice and to identify women in most need. While some areas are known to provide good prepregnancy care and advice for women with conditions such as type 1 and 2 diabetes and epilepsy, there is currently no arrangement in the region to ensure that women of childbearing age are given appropriate advice and support in a coordinated way.

Women with long-term conditions are usually followed up routinely in secondary care where opportunistic advice may be given by their specialists before embarking on pregnancy. A key challenge is to develop a clinical and commissioning model for the provision of prepregnancy care in the community with general practitioners at the forefront of this service provision. A conference is under way involving a wide range of stakeholders to identify the areas of prepregnancy care where models of care and commissioning can be developed. Pilot sites for developing these services will be identified. Quality standards will then be developed with the aim of implementing learning from the pilot projects. Lessons learned will help commissioners to purchase the service across the region. It is an ambitious project but is achievable, and will be a model of care that can be developed on a regional basis. Currently, no such innovative model exists at a regional level in the UK. The models of care will involve prepregnancy care for diabetes, obesity, epilepsy and maternal mental health.

Maternal mental health

When complex social and psychological needs are identified, there should be clear and robust pathways for the management of problems such as mental health and social needs. The midwife plays a key role in sign - posting the woman to the appropriate specialist services. To develop maternal mental health services across the region, the clinical programme board, together with the mental health clinical programme board, has been able to secure funding to deliver improving access to psychological therapies training to all maternity and neonatal staff, to raise awareness and support available to mothers during their pregnancy and following delivery of their babies.

Choice and normality of birth

All current guidelines recommend that the ideal intrapartum care path - way should provide:[3,8]

- normality of birth
- communication
- support for the mother, with one-to-one care in established labour
- choice of birth, home birth, midwife-led unit or obstetric unit.

To promote normality of birth, there should be an attempt to safely reduce interventions such as caesarean sections. The recommendations of *Maternity Matters* have been applied when developing such strategies.[3] These measures would include the following:

- increased use of midwife-led birthing units
- greater encouragement of home births
- policies to provide vaginal birth after caesarean section
- provision of external cephalic version for breech presentation.

These initiatives are being developed regionally and facilitated by the clinical programme board, working with provider maternity units and commissioners. The monitoring of performance is via the maternity dashboard, which is updated on a regular basis to provide units with information on their performance, allowing them to benchmark their progress against other units in the region.

As part of the choice and normality agenda, the clinical programme board has recommended that each acute trust will have a co-located midwife-led unit with clear pathways for transfer of care. The clinical programme board is working with commissioners to ensure that this target is met and there is a commitment from all units that this will be achieved by 2011.

Workforce

Standards for the midwifery workforce have been laid down in the *Safer Childbirth* document.[9] The recommended ratio of midwives to births (1/28 low-risk deliveries, 1/25 high-risk deliveries and one-to-one care in established labour) meant that extra staff resources would be required to achieve this standard. The clinical programme board recommended a more pragmatic solution of 1/30 as an average midwife-to-birth ratio, recognising that the ultimate standard all maternity units have to achieve are as stated in *Safer Childbirth*. This takes account of the current national shortage of midwives and the difficulties many units are facing with recruitment and retention.

There has been considerable collaboration between commissioners and provider units. Midwifery workforce numbers have significantly increased across the region with a 3-year recruitment and retention strategy. This increase in midwifery establishment is key to ensure the guarantee of one-to-one care in established labour, thereby improving outcome and satisfaction for mothers. The skill mix of the midwifery workforce is also being reviewed to ensure that the appropriate level of expertise is available in the maternity service so that midwives are able to fulfil their roles in a meaningful way. Together with the workforce directorate, the clinical programme board has been successful in procuring extra training places for student midwives and funding precep-torship programmes for newly qualified midwives. Training packages for supervisors of midwives have also been secured.

Clinical pathways

Uniformity of clinical pathways across the East of England region has been identified as being an important strand of providing consistent and high-quality care. Together with the mental health clinical programme board, the perinatal mental health pathway is being developed for the whole region.

A clinical pathway for the management of threatened preterm labour, involving bedside testing for fibronectin, has also been developed. The clinical programme board has succeeded in procuring the test on a regional basis, helping to keep costs down for units to adopt the test and pathway.

Neonatal care

A review of the neonatal cots in the region has been occurring in different districts within the East of England region. The ultimate aim is to increase the capacity of neonatal intensive cots and local special care cots but reduce the number of high-dependency care cots in the region, ensuring the right mix of cots for the needs of the region. Clear pathways for transfer of babies in and out have been drawn up. This, together with the improved transport service, should see a reduction of transfers of mothers and babies out of the region. The regional neonatal transport service is now available 24 hours a day, 7 days a week.

Safety, quality and patient experience

To monitor the quality of maternity services delivered across the region the clinical programme board, in discussion with commissioners and clinicians, has developed a maternity dashboard. This provides the opportunity to benchmark across the region each trust's quality indicators, ensuring that the services provided are safe and effective. It has also provided the opportunity to ensure that the reported data are robust and accurately reflect the activity undertaken, highlighting areas of good practice and those that require further support.

All units are encouraged to adopt the RCOG Clinical Dashboard to monitor safety and quality issues. Patient experience is monitored by surveys and in conjunction with the Patient Experience Board.

Key challenges

The key challenge to date has been that of clinical engagement. In particular, engaging clinicians in primary care has been difficult because of the ability of general practitioners to commit their time to the programme. The clinical programme board is working with PCTs and the practice-based commissioning groups of general practitioners to address this. Clinicians should be given the appropriate time and support to be engaged in such an important change agenda.

The significant challenge in the near future is the potential reduction and limitation of growth in funding for development of services. This is being addressed by the recently launched quality, innovation, prevention and productivity programme. The clinical programme board is currently examining the work streams to ensure that the initiatives are both affordable and able to deliver improvement without more investment than is currently projected.

Meeting the challenge

In any review of services and development of a clinical vision, it is vital that clinicians are placed at the forefront of developing the ideas and leading change. Clinical leaders from all fields were identified before the process and invited to participate. It is also equally important that there be strong user involvement so that the services developed are really what patients want and not just for clinicians. Good engagement with commissioners is also a recipe for success as they are the ones who will be commissioning services for the population.

Busy clinicians need to be provided with the time and support to lead the change. NHS East of England has recognised this and has invested in clinical leadership programmes for all clinical staff as they, not managers, will be at the helm of shaping future services.

A clear structure (Figure 21.1) needs to be identified so that there are clear lines of responsibility and accountability. Good evidence and robust data are crucial so that the right information can inform the development of strategic change. In this review, a clear structure has been set up with support from top management at board level and also clinicians at most levels:

- The clinical programme board reports to the *Towards the Best, Together* steering group, which in turn reports to the board of the SHA.
- The chair of the clinical programme board is a member of the East of England management board, which comprises the chief executives of all the primary care trusts and executive directors of the SHA.
- The programme lead meets the heads of midwifery monthly and maternity commissioners bimonthly, where a regular update on the progress of the clinical programme board is discussed. Joint heads of midwifery and maternity commissioner meetings also take place on a quarterly basis.
- There is a good engagement exercise whereby the chair and programme lead have undertaken a series of visits to provider trusts to discuss progress of the work of the clinical programme board with clinicians, senior managers and commissioners.
- Regular reports are taken to the directors of commissioning for discussion and agreement regarding the development of the metrics for delivery.

All the above measures ensure good communication at all levels.

Conclusion

The NHS has seen a major review in 2008–2010 to develop services that will be fit for purpose for the 21st century. This will be of significant benefit for the patient and the health of the nation. Clinicians have been

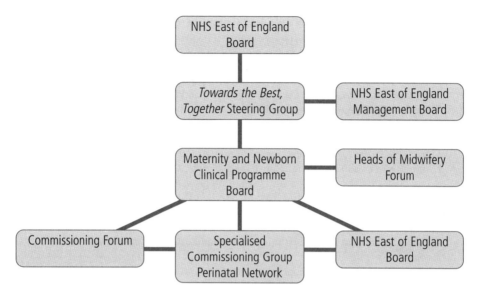

Figure 21.1 Reporting structure of the clinical programme board

placed at the forefront of the review, giving them the opportunity to shape the future of the NHS. This has truly been a clinically led and evidence-based exercise, developing high-quality care with the patient at the centre of the development.

References

1. Department of Health. *High Quality Care for All: NHS Next Stage Review Final Report*. Cm7432. London: The Stationery Office; 2008 [http://www.dh.gov.uk/en/publicationsandstatistics/publications/publicationspolicyandguidance/DH_085825].
2. NHS East of England. *Towards the Best, Together. A Clinical Vision for our NHS, Now and for the Next Decade*. Cambridge: NHS East of England; 2009 [http://www.eoe.nhs.uk/page.php?area_id=10].
3. Department of Health. *Maternity Matters: Choice, Access and Continuity of Care in a Safe Service*. London: DH; 2008 [http://www.dh.gov.uk/en/Publicationsand statistics/Publications/PublicationsPolicyAndGuidance/DH_073312].
4. Department of Health. *Our Health, Our Care, Our Say: A New Direction for Community Services*. London: HMSO; 2006 [http://www.dh.gov.uk/en/Publications andstatistics/Publications/PublicationsPolicyAndGuidance/DH_4127453].
5. Department of Health. *National Service Framework for Children, Young People and Maternity Services Standard 11: Maternity Services*. London: DH; 2004 [http://www.dh.gov.uk/en/Publicationsandstatistics/Publications/Publications PolicyAndGuidance/Browsable/DH_4094336].

6. National Institute for Health and Clinical Excellence. *Fertility: Assessment and Treatment for People With Fertility Problems*. Clinical guideline CG11. London: NICE; 2004 [http://guidance.nice.org.uk/CG11].

7. Lewis G, editor. *Saving Mothers' Lives: Reviewing Maternal Deaths to Make Motherhood Safer 2003–2005. The Seventh Report of the Confidential Enquiries into Maternal Deaths in the United Kingdom*. London: CEMACH; 2007 [http://www.cmace.org.uk/getdoc/319fb647-d2c6-4b47-b6a0-a853a2f4de1b/Maternal-1.aspx].

8. National Institute for Health and Clinical Excellence. *Intrapartum Care: Management and Delivery of Care to Women in Labour*. Clinical Guideline 55. London: NICE; 2007 [http://guidance.nice.org.uk/CG55].

9. Royal College of Obstetricians and Gynaecologists, Royal College of Anaesthetists, Royal College of Midwives and Royal College of Paediatrics and Child Health. *Safer Childbirth: Minimum Standards for the Organisation and Delivery of Care in Labour*. London; RCOG Press; 2007 [http://www.rcog.org.uk/womens-health/clinical-guidance/safer-childbirth-minimum-standards-organisation-and-delivery-care-la].

CHAPTER 22
Key indicators

Tahir Mahmood and Charnjit Dhillon

The RCOG published its document *Standards in Maternity Care* in 2008 and is being used widely by commissioners, providers and policy makers.[1] It sets out the principles of quality-assured maternity services. This section identifies some key indicators as exemplars, although we recommend that you make use of the whole document.

Strategy

✓ When developing a local maternity services strategy, involve all interested parties (patients, staff and commissioners) and take information from regulators and standard-setting bodies.

✓ Patients expect and value safety above everything else.

✓ When implementing change, form multidisciplinary teams around the processes that need changing and encourage those with expertise to step forward and become leaders.

Prepregnancy care for women with social needs

✓ Prepregnancy care for women with social needs is essential. It should promote social and physical stability and wellbeing before conception.

✓ Prepregnancy care can improve outcomes in high-risk pregnancies regardless of whether the high-risk status is of medical or social aetiology.

✓ Women who are socially disadvantaged do not seek advice through routine health channels. Multidisciplinary agencies already providing services for such women should be trained in needs assessment and delivery of basic components of prepregnancy care and should collaborate with reproductive healthcare services to ensure routine provision of prepregnancy care for all women with whom they are in contact.

Access to early pregnancy care

✓ Policies should be in place for the management of early pregnancy problems.

✓ Policies should be in place to meet the national target of booking women before 12 completed weeks of pregnancy.

✓ Strategies should be in place to identify women with pre-existing medical conditions.

✓ Strategies should be in place to identify socially disadvantaged women to develop individualised antenatal care.

✓ Effective communication strategies should be in place to support women who do not speak English to improve access to services.

Antenatal fetal abnormality screening

✓ From a public health perspective, the identification of anomalies can improve perinatal morbidity and mortality, as conditions may be identified early in pregnancy and managed accordingly.

✓ Specific measures must be taken to become risk-averse, as opposed to risk-reactive, by conforming to all elements of quality assurance: standards, defining roles and responsibilities, training, qualified and competent staff, audit and monitoring and using approved tools for the job.

Antenatal care for low-risk pregnancies

✓ Women should be encouraged to book early in their pregnancy.

✓ Antenatal care for women with a current low-risk pregnancy should be provided by a midwife.

✓ Antenatal screening should be offered in accordance with the National Screening Committee recommendations.

▣ Antenatal care for women with pre-existing medical, obstetric or mental health conditions

✓ A referral care pathway should be in place so that women are referred to high-risk clinics.

✓ A multidisciplinary team should be in place to provide care to women with previously known medical condition(s), according to agreed care plans.

✓ A fast-track care pathway should be in place within regional maternity networks for early referral to a specialist team for assessment.

✓ A care pathway should be in place in each region for routine and emergency situations in high-risk pregnancies.

✓ Perinatal networks should ensure that robust communication plans are in place between all professionals and the woman.

▣ Antenatal care for women developing medical or obstetric problems during pregnancy

✓ The majority of women experience no complications during pregnancy, but a significant proportion requires additional multidisciplinary care to maximise healthy outcomes.

✓ The provision of written patient information will aid in the understanding of conditions about which women will frequently have no prior knowledge.

✓ Recognised referral pathways must be established and accessible.

▣ Managing risk in antenatal care

✓ Managing risk in antenatal care is dependent on identification of risk factors through risk assessment. Women may move between low and high risk at different stages and risk management processes must ensure that they receive the level of care they need in an effective and safe manner.

✓ Significant risk issues include increasing obesity, pre-existing medical conditions, increasing maternal age, not speaking English, women who do not access care and vulnerable groups.

✓ Risk management should include organisational culture, risk assessment, training, induction, guidelines, communication, audit and learning from adverse incidents, claims and complaints.

Intrapartum care for low-risk pregnancies

✓ Wherever the birth takes place, the principles and practice will remain the same, but organisational and service infrastructures should be in place to support delivery of midwifery-led care for women assessed to be at 'low risk' in labour.

✓ A woman with a healthy pregnancy and spontaneous onset of labour should be afforded care that maintains this status.

✓ Teaching and training needs to emphasise the importance of recognising normal physiological progress of labour to avoid unnecessary medical interventions.

Intrapartum care for high-risk pregnancies

✓ Risk assessment of the woman and fetus prior to labour is essential.

✓ High-risk pregnancies should be delivered in a tertiary centre where multidisciplinary expertise is available.

✓ The views of women and healthcare providers should be taken into account when service development is contemplated.

Obesity in pregnancy

✓ Maternity services should develop a clinical care pathway for maternal obesity that takes into account locally agreed strategies for management.

✓ Dietetic services and weight management interventions should be developed based on local population needs.

✓ The local organisation has responsibility for ensuring that health professionals involved in maternity care have access to appropriate education and training related to maternal obesity.

Prevention of hypoxic ischaemic encephalopathy

✓ Current approaches for the prevention of hypoxic ischaemic encephalopathy include antenatal identification and monitoring of fetal growth restriction and electronic fetal monitoring accompanied by intrapartum fetal blood sampling.

✓ Intrapartum monitoring of the fetal heart rate remains the most commonly used tool for identification of an at-risk fetus and allows for timely intervention.

✓ All units should have a regular continuing programme of in-service training, including cardiotocograph interpretation, drills on emergency caesarean section and neonatal resuscitation.

Risk management on the labour ward

✓ Risk management should be system-based.

✓ There are emerging examples of risk management-led interventions to improve safety, such as the RCOG Maternity Dashboard.

Place of birth

✓ Genuine choice depends on the woman and her partner having adequate and appropriate evidence-based information, given at the correct time, to support their decision making.

✓ Providers and commissioners should ensure that appropriate clinical governance, including staffing levels and reliable processes for transfer to obstetric care where necessary, are in place, with due attention given to achieving a balance between choice and safety.

High-risk pregnancy and neonatal services

✓ A written and agreed postnatal plan should be outlined before birth; for example, parents should be advised that delivery should occur at a unit that can provide the appropriate level of neonatal care for anticipated gestation, birth weight and any neonatal complications.

✓ Mothers and babies should remain together unless there is a clear clinical indication for admission for enhanced care. The care of the baby must not be inappropriately invasive.

✓ Transitional care, where babies remain with their mother but may be monitored closely, is the ideal setting for babies in these circumstances.

Anaesthesia service provision for maternity services

✓ A duty anaesthetist should be immediately available for the delivery suite 24 hours a day.

✓ When obstetric units are so small or their workload so sporadic that provision of the basic minimum staffing levels is not cost-effective, consideration should be given to amalgamation with other local units.

✓ There should be an agreed system whereby the anaesthetist is given sufficient advance notice of all potential high-risk delivieries.

✓ All grades of anaesthetist who are on-call for the delivery suite but do not have regular sessions there should spend time in the delivery suite with one of the regular obstetric anaesthetic consultants.

Postnatal care

✓ The partnership between healthcare professionals and the woman built in the antenatal period requires further input in the postnatal period to empower the woman, such that she can go on to guard her own health and that of her new baby both physically and emotionally.

✓ Coordination of services in the postnatal period is made more difficult by the transfer of care between health professionals and clinical settings. This requires a robust local strategy that outlines the specific roles, places and timings of postnatal care provision. The central tenet is clear, written communication.

Supporting families who experience adverse outcomes during pregnancy

✓ There should be dedicated facilities for parents whose baby dies.

✓ All that parents take home with them are their memories. The staff who cared for them form a large part of those memories.

✓ There should be clear pathways between secondary and primary care teams to help ensure continuing care and support.

The maternity dashboard

✓ The maternity dashboard is primarily a tool to record maternity data in an 'at-a-glance' format to aid the clinical governance process.

✓ Use of existing data sources optimises the reliability of a dashboard and the speed and efficiency of production.

Commissioning for regional maternity services

✓ The design of the regional clinical service must be clinically led, with input from clinicians, users of the service and commissioners.

✓ Solutions must be evidence-based to develop high-quality care, with women at the centre of the development.

Index

Also available from RCOG Press

Let's do audit!

A practical guide to improving the quality of medical
care through criterion-based audit

This book is aimed at anyone who
wants to improve the quality of the
medical care they provide: nurses,
doctors, managers, healthcare
assistants, students, laboratory
technicians. It details a simple, free
and effective process for examining
the quality of the care you provide
through criterion-based audit: decide
what you should be doing in any
circumstance, examine whether or
not you are doing it, then look for
ways of improving your care until you
are doing it correctly.

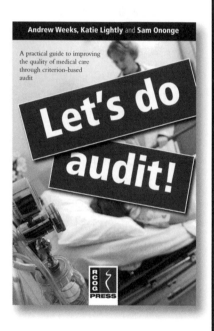

This book will be of interest to anyone in healthcare practice who is keen
to find a better way of working.

104 pages
ISBN 978-1-906985-35-6
£19.99 (£14.99 RCOG Fellows, Members and registered trainees)

www.rcogbookshop.com

Also available from RCOG Press

Models of Care
in Women's Health

This book aims to help clinicians improve the quality of care in gynaecological practice. In each area of practice covered, it addresses issues of clinical effectiveness, increasing patient expectations and service organisation, helping clinicians to take responsibility for developing services that meet women's needs as well as managing their individual medical conditions.

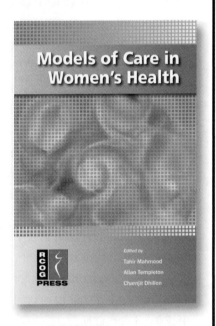

This book is of practical value for trainees, clinicians, managers and commissioners of services.

172 pages

ISBN 978-1-906985-18-9

£26 (£19.50 RCOG Fellows, Members and registered trainees)

www.rcogbookshop.com